ELSEVIER'S DICTIONARY OF PUBLIC HEALTH

ELSEVIER'S DICTIONARY OF PUBLIC HEALTH

IN SIX LANGUAGES

ENGLISH - FRENCH - SPANISH - ITALIAN - DUTCH
AND GERMAN

Compiled and arranged on
an English alphabetical basis by

NIC J.I. DEBLOCK

Beesd, The Netherlands

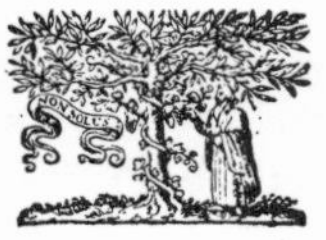

ELSEVIER SCIENTIFIC PUBLISHING COMPANY
Amsterdam — Oxford — New York 1976

ELSEVIER SCIENTIFIC PUBLISHING COMPANY
335 Jan van Galenstraat
P.O. Box 211, Amsterdam, The Netherlands

AMERICAN ELSEVIER PUBLISHING COMPANY, INC.
52 Vanderbilt Avenue
New York, New York 10017

ISBN: 0-444-41395-2

Printed in The Netherlands

FOREWORD

Increasing attention is being paid to the problems of health care in the various EEC countries, not only in the context of the Community itself but also on an international scale. One of the reasons for this is that much can be learned from the experience of other countries, as much from the difficulties and failures as from the successes. For all those who wish to acquaint themselves with the literature in this field, the frequently incomprehensible terminology is a significant obstacle. In the field of health care there are terms that are difficult to translate; these are in fact idioms. The same difficulties are encountered if one wishes to publish something in one of the frequently used international languages.

Mr. Deblock has collected a large number of terms in six languages and in this has done pioneering work. Naturally, as with any dictionary, you will not find every word or phrase you look for, and opinions may vary on the translation of a particular word. Similar words may have very different meanings in different languages, and in the field of health care this is related to the very complicated structures emerging from developments in the various countries. For this reason, it is very important for the author to receive reactions to his book so that the next edition, which will obviously be necessary, will comprise an even more extensive list of words.

Despite these inevitable reservations, I do believe that, with this book, an important aid to international communication and understanding has been created.

Prof.Dr. C.L.C. van Nieuwenhuizen

ABBREVIATIONS

f	feminine	f	Français
m	masculine	e	Español
n	neuter	i	Italiano
pl	plural	n	Nederlands
		d	Deutsch

ACKNOWLEDGEMENTS

The compilation of this dictionary would not have been possible without the assistance of others. My grateful thanks are due to:

Mr. Franco Noberasco, a medical student at the University of Genoa. He made it possible to add Italian to the five languages originally planned for, by taking charge of the Italian part of the dictionary.

Miss Suzan Meijer, who took care of much of the supporting work, such as the preparation of the indexes and the typing of the manuscript.

My wife, a qualified translator, who is now working in the health care field. She gave me valuable advice, revised the terminology and corrected the proofs.

Nic J.I. Deblock

BASIC TABLE

A

1 ABDOMINAL SURGERY
f chirurgie *f* abdominale
e cirugía *f* abdominal
i chirurgia *f* addominale
n buikchirurgie
d Abdominalchirurgie *f*

2 ABORTION
f avortement *m*
e aborto *m*
i aborto *m*
n abortus
d Abortus *m*

3 ABSENCE DUE TO SICKNESS;
ABSENTEEISM DUE TO SICKNESS;
MEDICAL ABSENTEEISM;
SICK ABSENTEEISM;
SICKNESS ABSENCE;
SICKNESS ABSENTEEISM
f absentéisme *m* médical
e ausencia *f* por enfermedad
i assenteismo *m* medico
n ziekteverzuim *n*
d Abwesenheit *f* infolge Krankheit

4 ABSENTEEISM DUE TO SICKNESS
see: ABSENCE DUE TO SICKNESS

5 ACADEMIC HOSPITAL;
TEACHING HOSPITAL;
UNIVERSITY HOSPITAL
f hôpital *m* académique;
centre *m* hospitalier universitaire;
hôpital *m* universitaire;
hôpital *m* d'université;
hôpital *m* d'enseignement
e hospital *m* académico;
hospital *m* universitario;
hospital *m* docente;
hospital *m* de enseñanza
i ospedale *m* universitario
n academisch ziekenhuis *n*;
universitair ziekenhuis *n*
d akademisches Krankenhaus *n*;
Universitätskrankenhaus *n*;
Unterrichtskrankenhaus *n*;
Ausbildungskrankenhaus *n*;
Lehrkrankenhaus *n*

6 ACCIDENT CARE
f soins *mpl* des accidentés
e cuidado *m* (atención *f*) de los accidentados
i cura *f* degli infortunati
n zorg voor ongevalspatiënten
d Unfallversorgung *f*

7 ACCIDENT CENTRE (CENTER)
f centre *m* pour accidentés
e centro *m* de accidentes;
centro *m* de accidentados
i centro *m* di ortopedia e traumatologia
n ongevallencentrum *n*
d Unfallzentrum *n*

8 ACCIDENT CLINIC
f clinique *f* pour accidentés;
clinique *f* traumatologique;
clinique *f* de traumatologie
e clínica *f* de accidentes;
clínica *f* de accidentados
i clinica *f* ortopedica e traumatologica
n ongevallenkliniek
d Unfallklinik *f*

9 ACCIDENT DEPARTMENT;
CASUALTY DEPARTMENT
f service *m* (département *m*) pour accidentés;
service *m* (département *m*) traumatologique;
service *m* (département *m*) de traumatologie
e servicio *m* (departamento *m*) de accidentes;
servicio *m* (departamento *m*) de accidentados
i divisione *f* di ortopedia e traumatologia
n ongevallenafdeling
d Unfallabteilung *f*

10 ACCIDENT HOSPITAL
f hôpital *m* pour accidentés
e hospital *m* de accidentes;
hospital *m* de accidentados
i ospedale *m* ortopedico e traumatologico
n ongevallenziekenhuis *n*
d Unfallkrankenhaus *n*

11 ACCIDENT INSURANCE
f assurance-accidents *f*;
assurance *f* contre les accidents
e seguro *m* de accidentes;
seguro *m* contra los accidentes
i assicurazione *f* contro gli incidenti
n ongevallenverzekering
d Unfallversicherung *f*

12 ACCIDENT PREVENTION
f prévention *f* des accidents
e prevención *f* de accidentes
i prevenzione *f* degli incidenti
n voorkomen *n* van ongevallen;
ongevallenbescherming
d Unfallverhütung *f*

13 ACCIDENT SERVICES;
CASUALTY SERVICES
f services *mpl* pour accidentés;
services *mpl* de soins aux accidentés;
services *mpl* traumatologiques;
services *mpl* de traumatologie
e servicios *mpl* de accidentes;
servicios *mpl* de accidentados
i servizi *mpl* di ortopedia e traumatologia
n ongevallenvoorzieningen;
ongevallendiensten
d Unfalldienste *mpl*

14 ACCIDENT TREATMENT;
CASUALTY TREATMENT
f traitement *m* des accidentés
e tratamiento *m* de los accidentados
i trattamento *m* dei traumatizzati
n behandeling van ongevalspatiënten
d Unfallbehandlung *f*

15 ACUTE CARE
f soins *mpl* aigus

e cuidado *m* agudo;
atención *f* aguda
i cure *fpl* acute
n acute zorg
d Behandlung *f* akuter Fälle

16 ACUTE DISEASE
f maladie *f* aiguë
e enfermedad *f* aguda
i malattia *f* acuta
n acute ziekte
d akute Krankheit *f*

17 ACUTE HOSPITAL
f hôpital *m* de soins aigus;
hôpital *m* pour malades aigus
e hospital *m* para agudos
i ospedale *m* per malati acuti
n algemeen ziekenhuis *n*;
ziekenhuis *n* voor acute gevallen
d Akutkrankenhaus *n*

18 ACUTELY ILL PATIENT;
ACUTE PATIENT
f malade *m* (patient *m*) aigu
e paciente *m* (enfermo *m*) agudo
i malato *m* acuto
n acute patiënt
d Akutkranker *m*;
akut Erkrankter *m*

19 ACUTE PATIENT
see: ACUTELY ILL PATIENT

20 ADAPTED LAVATORY
f toilette *f* adaptée
e tocador *m* adaptado
i gabinetto *m* adattato
n aangepast toilet *n*
d angepasste Toilette *f*

21 ADMISSION;
INPATIENT ADMISSION
f admission *f*;
entrée *f*
e admisión *f*;
ingreso *m*
i accettazione *f*;
entrata *f*
n opneming;
opname
d Aufnahme *f*

22 ADMISSION AGREEMENT;
ADMISSION CONTRACT
f contrat *m* d'admission
e contrato *m* de admisión
i contratto *m* d'accettazione
n opname-overeenkomst
d Aufnahmevertrag *m*

23 ADMISSION CONTRACT
see: ADMISSION AGREEMENT

24 ADMISSION DEPARTMENT;
ADMISSION SERVICE
f service *m* (département *m*) des admissions
e servicio *m* (departamento *m*) de admisión
i servizio *m* di accettazione
n opname-afdeling
d Aufnahmeabteilung *f*;
Aufnahmedienst *m*

25 ADMISSION EXAMINATION
f examen *m* d'admission
e examen *m* de admisión
i visita *f* preliminare
n opname-onderzoek *n*
d Aufnahmeuntersuchung *f*

26 ADMISSION INDEX;
ADMISSION RATE
f taux *m* des admissions;
indice *m* d'hospitalisation
e índice *m* de admisión;
tasa *f* de admisión;
índice *m* de hospitalización;
tasa *f* de hospitalización
i tasso *m* delle accettazioni;
tasso *m* di ospedalizzazione;
indice *m* di ospedalizzazione
n opname-index;
opnamefrequentie
d Krankenhaushäufigkeit *f*

27 ADMISSION OFFICE
f bureau *m* des admissions
e oficina *f* de admisión
i ufficio *m* dell' accettazione
n opname-administratie
d Aufnahmebüro *n*

28 ADMISSION RATE
see: ADMISSION INDEX

29 ADMISSION SERVICE
see: ADMISSION DEPARTMENT

30 ADMISSION STATISTICS
f statistique *f* des admissions
e estadística *f* de admisiones
i statistica *f* delle ammissioni
n opnamestatistiek
d Aufnahmestatistik *f*

31 ADMISSION UNIT
f unité *f* d'admission
e unidad *f* de admisión
i unità *f* di accettazione
n opname-eenheid
d Aufnahmestation *f*

32 AEROTHERAPY
f aérothérapie *f*
e aeroterapia *f*
i aeroterapia *f*
n aerotherapie
d Aerotherapie *f*

33 AFFILIATED HOSPITAL
f hôpital *m* lié
e hospital *m* afiliado;
hospital *m* de afiliación
i ospedale *m* aggregato
n geaffilieerd ziekenhuis *n*
d Nicht-Universitätskrankenhaus *n* als Ausbildungsstätte für Medizinstudenten

34 AFFILIATION
f affiliation *f*
e afiliación *f*
i aggregazione *f*
n affiliatie
d Funktionieren *n* eines Nicht-Universitätskrankenhauses als Ausbildungsstätte für Medizinstudenten

35 AFTER CARE
f post-cure *f*;
surveillance *f* de post-cure
e cuidado *m* posterior;
asistencia *f* posterior;
vigilancia *f* postcura;
atención *f* postcura
i assistenza *f* post-ospedaliera
n nazorg
d Nachsorge *f*;
Nachpflege *f*;
nachgehende Fürsorge *f*

36 AFTER CARE CENTRE (CENTER)
f centre *m* de post-cure;
foyer *m* de post-cure;
dispensaire *m* de post-cure
e centro *m* de cuidado posterior
i centro *m* di assistenza post-ospedaliera;
ambulatorio *m* di assistenza post-ospedaliera
n nazorgcentrum *n*
d Nachsorgestelle *f*;
Nachsorgeanstalt *f*

37 AFTER CARE HOSPITAL
f établissement *m* de post-cure
e hospital *m* de cuidado posterior
i poliambulatorio *m* per l'assistenza post-ospedaliera
n nazorgziekenhuis *n*
d Nachsorgeklinik *f*

38 AFTER CARE PATIENT
f malade *m* (patient *m*) recevant des soins post-hospitaliers
e paciente *m* (enfermo *m*) que recibe cuidado posterior
i malato *m* che usufruisce di assistenza post-ospedaliera
n nazorgpatiënt
d Nachsorgepatient *m*

39 AFTER TREATMENT
f traitement *m* consécutif
e tratamiento *m* ulterior;
apoterapia *f*
i trattamento *m* post-espedaliero dei dimessi
n nabehandeling
d Nachbehandlung *f*

40 AIDE;
ASSISTANT NURSE;
AUXILIARY;
AUXILIARY NURSE;
NURSE AIDE;
NURSING ASSISTANT;
NURSING AUXILIARY
f aide-infirmière *f*;
aide-soignante *f*;
infirmière *f* assistante;
infirmière *f* auxiliaire;
garde-malade *f* auxiliaire
e ayudante *f* de enfermería;
enfermera *f* auxiliar;
auxiliar *f*;
auxiliar *f* de enfermería
i aiuto-infermiera *f*;
infermiera *f* ausiliaria;
ausiliaria *f*
n verpleeghulp
d Hilfspflegerin *f*;
Hilfsschwester *f*;
Krankenpflegehelferin *f*;
Krankenpflegehilfe *f*;
Pflegehelferin *f*;
Pflegehilfskraft *f*;
Schwesternhelferin *f*;
Schwesternhilfe *f*

41 AIR LOCK;
BED STERILIZING ROOM;
LIGHT LOCK
f sas *m* pour lits
e esclusa *f* para camas
i camera *f* di disinfezione per letti
n bedsluis;
beddensluis
d Bettenschleuse *f*

42 AIR POLLUTION
f pollution *f* aérienne;
pollution *f* de l'air
e ensuciamiento *m* del aire
i inquinamento *m* atmosferico
n luchtvervuiling;
luchtverontreiniging
d Luftverschmutzung *f*

43 ALLERGIC DISEASE
f maladie *f* allergique
e enfermedad *f* alérgica
i malattia *f* di natura allergica
n allergische ziekte
d allergische Krankheit *f*

44 ALLERGIST
f allergiste *m*
e alergista *m*
i allergologo *m*
n allergoloog
d Allergologe *m*

45 ALLERGY
f allergie *f*
e alergia *f*
i allergia *f*
n allergie
d Allergie *f*

46 AMBULANCE;
AMBULANCE CAR
f ambulance *f*;
auto *f* d'ambulance
e ambulancia *f*;
coche *m* ambulancia;
automóvil *m* de sanidad
i ambulanza *f*
n ambulance;
ziekenauto
d Ambulanz *f*;
Krankenwagen *m*

47 AMBULANCE CAR
see: AMBULANCE

48 AMBULANCE ENTRANCE
f entrée *f* des ambulances
e entrada *f* de las ambulancias
i entrata *f* delle ambulanze
n ambulance-ingang
d Ambulanzeingang *m*

49 AMBULANCE HALL
f hall *m* des ambulances
e hall *m* de las ambulancias
i hall *f* delle ambulanze

n ambulancehal
d Ambulanzhalle *f*

50 AMBULANCE PERSONNEL
f personnel *m* ambulancier
e personal *m* de ambulancia
i personale *m* addetto all'ambulanza
n ambulancepersoneel *n*
d Ambulanzpersonal *n*

51 AMBULANCE SERVICE
f service *m* ambulancier;
service *m* d'ambulance
e servicio *m* de ambulancia
i servizio *m* d'ambulanza
n ambulancedienst
d Ambulanzdienst *m*

52 AMBULANCE TRANSPORT
f transport *m* par ambulance
e transporte *m* por ambulancia
i trasporto *m* mediante ambulanza
n ambulancevervoer *n*
d Ambulanztransport *m*;
Krankenwagentransport *m*

53 AMBULANT CARE;
AMBULATORY CARE;
OUTPATIENT CARE
f soins *mpl* ambulatoires;
soins *mpl* ambulants;
soins *mpl* externes
e cuidado *m* ambulatorio;
atención *f* ambulatoria
i cure *fpl* ambulatoriali
n poliklinische zorg;
ambulante zorg
d ambulante Fürsorge *f*;
ambulante Pflege *f*;
ambulante Betreuung *f*;
ambulante Versorgung *f*

54 AMBULANT HEALTH CARE;
AMBULATORY HEALTH CARE;
OUTPATIENT HEALTH CARE
f soins *mpl* sanitaires ambulatoires;
soins *mpl* sanitaires ambulants;
soins *mpl* sanitaires externes
e cuidado *m* sanitario ambulatorio;
atención *f* sanitaria ambulatoria
i cure *fpl* sanitarie ambulatoriali
n poliklinische gezondheidszorg;
ambulante gezondheidszorg
d ambulante Gesundheitsfürsorge *f*;
ambulante Gesundheitspflege *f*;
ambulante Krankenfürsorge *f*

55 AMBULANT INPATIENT
f malade *m* (patient *m*) hospitalisé ambulant
e paciente *m* (enfermo *m*) hospitalizado ambulante
i malato *m* ospedalizzato in grado di alzarsi
n ambulante klinische patiënt
d ambulanter stationärer Patient *m*

56 AMBULANT OUTPATIENT
f malade *m* (patient *m*) externe ambulant
e paciente *m* (enfermo *m*) externo ambulante
i malato *m* esterno in grado di alzarsi
n ambulante poliklinische patiënt
d ambulanter Poliklinikpatient *m*

57 AMBULANT PATIENT
f malade *m* (patient *m*) ambulant
e paciente *m* (enfermo *m*) ambulante
i malato *m* in grado di alzarsi
n ambulante patiënt
d ambulanter Patient *m* (Kranker *m*)

58 AMBULATORY CARE
see: AMBULANT CARE

59 AMBULATORY CARE SERVICES;
AMBULATORY SERVICES;
OUTPATIENT SERVICES;
POLYCLINICAL SERVICES
f services *mpl* des consultations externes;
services *mpl* externes;
services *mpl* polycliniques;
services *mlp* ambulatoires;
services *mpl* de soins ambulatoires
e servicios *mpl* ambulatorios;
servicios *mpl* de pacientes externos
i servizi *mpl* di cure ambulatoriali;
consulti *mpl* e cure esterni
n poliklinische voorzieningen;
voorzieningen voor ambulante zorg
d ambulante Dienste *mpl*;
Dienste *mpl* für ambulante und poliklinische Behandlung

60 AMBULATORY CONSULTATION;
OUTPATIENT CONSULTATION;
POLYCLINICAL CONSULTATION
f consultation *f* externe;
consultation *f* ambulatoire
e consulta *f* ambulatoria;
consulta *f* externa
i consulto *m* ambulatoriale;
consulto *m* esterno
n poliklinisch consult *n*
d poliklinische Konsultation *f*;
ambulante Konsultation *f*

61 AMBULATORY HEALTH CARE
see: AMBULANT HEALTH CARE

62 AMBULATORY PATIENT;
HOSPITAL OUTPATIENT;
OUTPATIENT
f malade *m* (patient *m*) ambulatoire;
malade *m* (patient *m*) externe;
malade *m* (patient *m*) extérieur;
consultant *m* externe
e paciente *m* (enfermo *m*) ambulatorio;
paciente *m* (enfermo *m*) externo
i malato *m* ambulatoriale;
malato *m* esterno
n poliklinische patiënt
d Poliklinikpatient *m*

63 AMBULATORY SERVICES
see: AMBULATORY CARE SERVICES

64 AMBULATORY TREATMENT;
OUTPATIENT TREATMENT;
POLYCLINICAL TREATMENT
f traitement *m* ambulatoire
e tratamiento *m* ambulatorio
i trattamento *m* ambulatoriale
n poliklinische behandeling;
ambulante behandeling
d ambulante Behandlung *f*;
Poliklinikbehandlung *f*

65 ANATOMICAL PATHOLOGY
f anatomie *f* pathologique
e anatomía *f* patológica
i anatomia *f* patologica
n pathologische anatomie
d pathologische Anatomie *f*

66 ANATOMIST
f anatomiste *m*
e anatomista *m*
i anatomico *m*
n anatoom
d Anatomiker *m*

67 ANATOMY
f anatomie *f*
e anatomía *f*
i anatomia *f*
n anatomie
d Anatomie *f*

68 ANESTHESIA;
ANESTHETICS
f anesthésie *f*
e anestesia *f*
i anestesia *f*
n anesthesie
d Anästhesie *f*

69 ANESTHESIA APPARATUS
f appareils *mpl* d'anesthésie
e aparatos *mpl* de anestesia
i apparecchi *mpl* d'anestesia
n anesthesie-apparatuur
d Anästhesiegeräte *npl*;
Narkosegeräte *npl*

70 ANESTHESIA DEPARTMENT;
ANESTHESIOLOGY DEPARTMENT
f service *m* (département *m*) d'anesthésie
e servicio *m* (departamento *m*) de anestesia
i servizio *m* di anestesia
n anesthesie-afdeling
d Anästhesie-Abteilung *f*

71 ANESTHESIA NURSE;
NURSE-ANESTHETIST
f infirmière *f* anesthésiste
e enfermera *f* anestetista
i infermiera *f* anestesista
n anesthesie-verpleegkundige;
verpleegkundige voor narcosewerkzaamheden
d Anästhesieschwester *f*;
Narkoseschwester *f*

72 ANESTHESIA-RESUSCITATION DEPARTMENT
f service *m* (département *m*) d'anesthésie-réanimation
e servicio *m* (departamento *m*) de anestesia y reanimación;
servicio *m* (departamento *m*) de anestesia y resucitación
i servizio *m* di anestesia e di rianimazione
n anesthesie- en reanimatie-afdeling
d Anästhesie- und Wiederbelebungsabteilung *f*;
Anästhesie- und Reanimationsabteilung

73 ANESTHESIOLOGIST
f anesthésiste *m*
e anestetista *m*
i anestesista *m*
n anesthesist
d Anästhesist *m*

74 ANESTHESIOLOGY
f anesthésiologie *f*
e anestesiología *f*
i anestesiologia *f*
n anesthesiologie
d Anästhesiologie *f*

75 ANESTHESIOLOGY DEPARTMENT
see: ANESTHESIA DEPARTMENT

76 ANESTHETIC ROOM
f salle *f* d'anesthésie
e sala *f* de anestesia
i sala *f* d'anestesia
n anesthesiekamer
d Anästhesieraum *m*

77 ANESTHETICS
see: ANESTHESIA

78 ANIMAL EXPERIMENTATION
f expérimentation *f* animale
e experimentación *f* con animales
i sperimentazione *f* sugli animali
n experiment *n* op dieren
d Tierversuch *m*

79 ANTI-CANCER CENTRE (CENTER);
CANCER CENTRE (CENTER)
f centre *m* anticancéreux;
centre *m* de lutte contre le cancer
e consultorio *m* anticanceroso
i centro *m* antitumorale;
centro *m* oncologico
n kankercentrum *n*;
consultatiebureau *n* voor kankerbestrijding
d Krebsberatungsstelle *f*

80 ANTISEPTIC TECHNIQUES
f techniques *fpl* antiseptiques
e técnicas *fpl* antisépticas
i tecniche *fpl* antisettiche
n antiseptische technieken
d antiseptische Techniken *fpl*

81 APPOINTMENT SYSTEM
f système *m* des rendez-vous
e sistema *m* de citas
i sistema *m* di visita mediante appuntamento
n afspraaksysteem *n*
d Verabredungssystem *n*

82 AREA PER BED
f surface *f* par lit
e superficie *f* por cama
i spazio *m* per posto-letto
n oppervlakte per bed
d Flache *f* pro Bett

83 ARMED FORCES HOSPITAL;
ARMY HOSPITAL;
MILITARY HOSPITAL
f hôpital *m* militaire
e hospital *m* militar;
hospital *m* del ejército
i ospedale *m* militare
n militair ziekenhuis *n*;
militair hospitaal *n*
d Militärkrankenhaus *n*;
Lazarett *n*

84 ARMY HOSPITAL
see: ARMED FORCES HOSPITAL

85 ARTIFICIAL DENTURE;
ARTIFICIAL TEETH
f dents *mpl* artificiels;
prothèse *f* dentaire
e dientes *mpl* postizos;
prótesis *f* dentaria
i protesi *f* dentaria
n kunstgebit *n*;
mondprothese
d Zahnersatz *m*;
Zahnprothese *f*

86 ARTIFICIAL HEART
f coeur *m* artificiel
e corazón *m* artificial
i cuore *m* artificiale
n kunsthart *n*
d künstliches Herz *n*

87 ARTIFICIAL INSEMINATION
f insémination *f* artificielle
e inseminación *f* artificial
i fecondazione *f* artificiale
n kunstmatige inseminatie;
kunstmatige bevruchting
d künstliche Befruchtung *f*

88 ARTIFICIAL KIDNEY
f rein *m* artificiel
e riñón *m* artificial
i rene *m* artificiale
n kunstnier
d künstliche Niere *f*

89 ARTIFICIAL LIMBS
f membres *mpl* artificiels
e miembros *mpl* artificiales
i arti *mpl* artificiali;
membra *fpl* artificiali
n kunstledematen
d Kunstglieder *npl*;
künstliche Glieder *npl*

90 ARTIFICIAL RESPIRATION
f respiration *f* artificielle
e respiración *f* artificial
i respirazione *f* artificiale
n kunstmatige ademhaling
d künstliche Atmung *f*

91 ARTIFICIAL TEETH
see: ARTIFICIAL DENTURE

92 ART THERAPY
f thérapie *f* de l'art
e terapia *f* del arte
i terapia *f* mediante l'arte
n kunsttherapie
d Kunsttherapie *f*

93 ASEPSIS
f asepsie *f*
e asepsia *f*
i asepsi *f*
n asepsis
d Asepsis *f*

94 ASEPTIC ROOM
f chambre *f* aseptique
e sala *f* aséptica
i camera *f* asettica
n aseptische ruimte
d aseptischer Raum *m*

95 ASEPTIC TECHNIQUES
f techniques *fpl* aseptiques
e técnicas *fpl* asépticas
i tecniche *fpl* asettiche
n aseptische technieken
d aseptische Techniken *fpl*

96 ASSISTANT NURSE
see: AIDE

97 ASTHMATIC CLINIC
f clinique *f* pour asthmatiques
e clínica *f* para asmáticos
i clinica *f* per asmatici
n astmakliniek
d Asthmaklinik *f*

98 ATTENDANT;
MALE NURSE;
NURSE
f infirmier *m*;
infirmière *f*;
garde-malade *m/f*
e enfermero *m*;
enfermera *f*
i infermiere *m*;
infermiera *f*
n verpleger;
verpleegster;
verpleegkundige;
algemeen verpleegkundige;
verplegende;
ziekenverzorgster;
verzorgster
d Krankenpfleger *m*;
Krankenpflegerin *f*;
Pfleger *m*;
Pflegerin *f*;
Krankenschwester *f*

99 ATTENDING PERSONNEL
f personnel *m* soignant
e personal *m* que atiende
i personale *m* curante
n behandelend personeel *n*
d Versorgungspersonal *n*

100 ATTENDING PHYSICIAN
f médecin *m* traitant
e médico *m* que atiende
i medico *m* curante
n behandelend arts
d behandlender Arzt *m*

101 AUDIOLOGIC CENTRE (CENTER)
f centre *m* d'audiologie
e centro *m* auditivo
i centro *m* d'audiologia
n audiologisch centrum *n*
d audiologisches Zentrum *n*

102 AUDIOLOGIST
f audiologiste *m*
e audiólogo *m*
i audiologo *m*
n audioloog
d Audiologe *m*

103 AUDIOLOGY
f audiologie *f*
e audiología *f*
i audiologia *f*
n audiologie
d Audiologie *f*

104 AUDIOMETRY
f audiométrie *f*
e audiometría *f*
i audiometria *f*
n audiometrie
d Audiometrie *f*

105 AUDIOMETRY ROOM
f salle *f* d'audiométrie
e sala *f* audiométrica
i sala *f* d'audiometria
n audiometriekamer
d Raum *m* für Audiometrie

106 AUTOCLAVE
f autoclave *m*
e autoclave *m*
i autoclave *f*
n autoclaaf
d Autoklav *m*

107 AUTOPSY;
NECROPSY;
NECROSCOPY;
POST-MORTEM EXAMINATION
f autopsie *f*;
nécropsie *f*
e autopsia *f*;
necroscopia *f*;
necropsia *f*
i autopsia *f*;
necropsia *f*
n autopsie;
lijkschouwing;
sectie
d Autopsie *f*;
Leichenschau *f*;
Obduktion *f*;
Sektion *f*

108 AUTOPSY ROOM;
POST-MORTEM ROOM
f salle *f* d'autopsie
e sala *f* de autopsia
i sala *f* d'autopsia
n sectiekamer
d Prosektur *f*;
Sektionsraum *m*

109 AUXILIARY
see: AIDE

110 AUXILIARY NURSE
see: AIDE

111 AUXILIARY NURSING PERSONNEL
f personnel *m* soignant auxiliaire
e personal *m* auxiliar de enfermería
i personale *m* curante ausiliario
n verplegend hulppersoneel *n*
d Hilfspflegepersonal *n*

112 AVERAGE DURATION OF HOSPITALIZATION;
AVERAGE DURATION OF HOSPITAL STAY;
AVERAGE DURATION OF INPATIENT HOSPITALIZATION;
AVERAGE DURATION OF STAY;
AVERAGE HOSPITALIZATION LENGTH;
AVERAGE HOSPITALIZATION TIME;
AVERAGE LENGTH OF HOSPITALIZATION;
AVERAGE LENGTH OF STAY;
AVERAGE STAY LENGTH
f durée *f* moyenne de l'hospitalisation;
durée *f* moyenne de séjour
e duración *f* media de la hospitalización;
duración *f* media de la estancia (estadía);
promedio *m* de la estancia (estadía)
i durata *f* media del soggiorno
n gemiddelde verpleegduur;
gemiddelde ligduur;
gemiddelde verblijfsduur;
gemiddelde opnameduur
d durchschnittliche Verweildauer *f*;
durchschnittliche Pflegedauer *f*;
durchschnittliche Aufenthaltsdauer *f*;
durchschnittliche Liegedauer *f*;
durchschnittliche Liegezeit *f*

113 AVERAGE DURATION OF HOSPITAL STAY
see: AVERAGE DURATION OF HOSPITALIZATION

114 AVERAGE DURATION OF INPATIENT HOSPITALIZATION
see: AVERAGE DURATION OF HOSPITALIZATION

115 AVERAGE DURATION OF STAY
see: AVERAGE DURATION OF HOSPITALIZATION

116 AVERAGE HOSPITALIZATION LENGTH
see: AVERAGE DURATION OF HOSPITALIZATION

117 AVERAGE HOSPITALIZATION TIME
see: AVERAGE DURATION OF HOSPITALIZATION

118 AVERAGE LENGTH OF HOSPITALIZATION
see: AVERAGE DURATION OF HOSPITALIZATION

119 AVERAGE LENGTH OF STAY
see: AVERAGE DURATION OF HOSPITALIZATION

120 AVERAGE STAY LENGTH
see: AVERAGE DURATION OF HOSPITALIZATION

B

121 BABY LINEN
f linge *m* pour nourrissons
e ropa *f* para nenes
i biancheria *f* per neonati
n babylinnen *n*
d Säuglingswäsche *f*

122 BACTERIAL DISEASE
f maladie *f* bactériologique
e enfermedad *f* bacteriológica
i malattia *f* batteriologica
n bacteriologische ziekte
d bakteriologische Krankheit *f*

123 BACTERIOLOGICAL LABORATORY;
BACTERIOLOGY LABORATORY
f laboratoire *m* bactériologique;
laboratoire *m* de bactériologie
e laboratorio *m* bacteriológico;
laboratorio *m* de bacteriología
i laboratorio *m* batteriologico;
laboratorio *m* di batteriologia
n bacteriologisch laboratorium *n*
d bakteriologisches Laboratorium *n*;
Laboratorium *n* für Bakteriologie

124 BACTERIOLOGICAL-SEROLOGICAL
LABORATORY
f laboratoire *m* de bactériologie et sérologie
e laboratorio *m* de bacteriología y serología
i laboratorio *m* di batteriologia e sierologia
n bacteriologisch-serologisch laboratorium *n*
d Laboratorium *n* für Bakteriologie und Serologie

125 BACTERIOLOGY
f bactériologie *f*
e bacteriología *f*
i batteriologia *f*
n bacteriologie
d Bakteriologie *f*

126 BACTERIOLOGY LABORATORY
see: BACTERIOLOGICAL LABORATORY

127 BALNEOTHERAPY
f balnéothérapie *f*
e balneoterapia *f*
i balneoterapia *f*
n balneotherapie
d Balneotherapie *f*;
Bädertherapie *f*

128 BANDAGE
f bandage *m*
e braguero *m*
i fasciatura *f*
n bandage
d Bandage *f*

129 BASIC CARE;
PRIMARY CARE
f soins *mpl* de base;
soins *mpl* élémentaires
e cuidado *m* de base
i cure *fpl* di base
n basisverzorging
d Grundversorgung *f*

130 BASIC HEALTH SERVICES
f services *mpl* sanitaires de base;
services *mpl* de santé de base
e servicios *mpl* sanitarios de base;
servicios *mpl* de salud de base;
servicios *mpl* de sanidad de base
i servizi *mpl* sanitari di base
n basisgezondheidszorg
d Grundgesundheitsdienste *mpl*;
Grundgesundheitswesen *n*

131 BASIC HOSPITAL
f hôpital *m* de base
e hospital *m* de base
i ospedale *m* generale zonale
n basisziekenhuis *n*
d Krankenhaus *n* für Grundversorgung

132 BASIC HOSPITAL CARE
f soins *mpl* hospitaliers de base;
soins *mpl* hospitaliers élémentaires
e cuidado *m* hospitalario de base;
atención *f* hospitalaria de base;
asistencia *f* hospitalaria de base
i assistenza *f* ospedaliera di base
n basisziekenhuisverzorging
d Grundversorgung *f* in einem Krankenhaus

133 BASIC NURSING CARE
f soins *mpl* infirmiers de base;
soins *mpl* infirmiers élémentaires
e enfermería *f* de base
i cure *fpl* infermieristiche di base
n basisverpleging
d Grundkrankenpflege *f*

134 BATH STRETCHER
f brancard *m* pour le bain
e camilla *f* para el baño
i barella *f* da bagno
n badbrancard
d Badebahre *f*

135 BED CAPACITY
f capacité *f* en lits;
capacité *f* des lits
e capacidad *f* de camas
i capacità *f* dei letti
n bedcapaciteit
d Bettenkapazität *f*

136 BED CENTRE (CENTER);
CENTRAL BED SUPPLY
f centrale *f* des lits
e central *f* de camas
i centrale *f* dei letti
n beddencentrale
d Bettenzentrale *f*

137 BED CLEANING CENTRE (CENTER);
CENTRAL BED CLEANING DEPARTMENT
f centrale *f* de nettoyage des lits;
service *m* central de nettoyage des lits
e central *f* de limpieza de camas;
servicio *m* central de limpieza de camas
i centrale *f* di pulizia letti
n centrale beddenreiniging;

centrale beddenreinigingsafdeling
d zentrale Bettenreinigung *f*;
zentrale Bettenreinigungsabteilung *f*

138 BED COMPLEMENT;
BED COUNT
f nombre *m* des lits
e número *m* de camas
i numero *m* di letti
n aantal *n* bedden;
beddenbestand *n*
d Bettenzahl *f*;
Bettenbestand *m*

139 BED COUNT
see: BED COMPLEMENT

140 BED DENSITY
f densité *f* des lits
e densidad *f* de camas
i densità *f* dei letti
n beddichtheid
d Bettendichte *f*

141 BED DISINFECTION
f désinfection *f* des lits
e desinfección *f* de camas
i disinfezione *f* dei letti
n beddesinfectie
d Bettendesinfektion *f*

142 BED DISTRIBUTION
f répartition *f* des lits
e distribución *f* de las camas
i spartizione *f* dei letti
n beddenverdeling
d Bettenaufteilung *f*

143 BED ELEVATOR;
BED LIFT
f monte-lits *m*
e ascensor *m* de camas
i ascensore *m* per il trasporto dei letti
n beddenlift
d Bettenaufzug *m*

144 BED LIFT
see: BED ELEVATOR

145 BED NEED;
BED REQUIREMENT;
DEMAND FOR BEDS
f besoin *m* en lits
e necesidad *f* de camas
i fabbisogno *m* di letti
n beddenbehoefte
d Bettenbedarf *m*

146 BED OCCUPANCY;
BED OCCUPATION
f occupation *f* des lits
e ocupación *f* de camas
i occupazione *f* dei letti
n bedbezetting
d Bettenbelegung *f*

147 BED OCCUPANCY PERCENT(AGE);
BED OCCUPANCY RATE;
BED OCCUPANCY RATIO;
BED OCCUPATION PERCENT(AGE);
BED OCCUPATION RATE;
BED OCCUPATION RATIO
f pourcentage *m* d'occupation des lits;
taux *m* d'occupation des lits
e porcentaje *m* de ocupación de camas;
tasa *f* de ocupación de camas
i percentuale *f* dei letti occupati;
tasso *m* d'occupazione dei letti
n bedbezettingspercentage *n*;
bedbezettingsgraad
d prozentuale Bettenbelegung *f*;
Bettenbelegungsprozentsatz *m*;
Bettenbelegungsgrad *m*

148 BED OCCUPANCY RATE
see: BED OCCUPANCY PERCENT

149 BED OCCUPANCY RATIO
see: BED OCCUPANCY PERCENT

150 BED OCCUPATION
see: BED OCCUPANCY

151 BED OCCUPATION PERCENT(AGE)
see: BED OCCUPANCY PERCENT

152 BED OCCUPATION RATE
see: BED OCCUPANCY PERCENT

153 BED OCCUPATION RATIO
see: BED OCCUPANCY PERCENT

154 BED PAN
f bassin *m* de lit;
vase *m* de lit;
vase *m* plat
e silleta *f*;
galanga *f*;
chata *f*
i padella *f*
n bedpan;
ondersteek;
steekbekken *n*;
steekpan
d Steckbecken *n*;
Stechbecken *n*;
Bettschüssel *f*;
Unterschieber *m*

155 BED PAN CLEANING APPARATUS
f appareil *m* à laver les bassins de lit
e aparato *m* para limpiar silletas
i apparecchio *m* per lavare le padelle
n bedpanreiniger
d Steckbeckenspülgerät *n*

156 BED PATIENT;
HOSPITAL INPATIENT;
HOSPITALIZED PATIENT;
INPATIENT
f malade *m* (patient *m*) hospitalisé;
hospitalisé *m*
e paciente *m* (enfermo *m*) hospitalizado;
paciente *m* (enfermo *m*) internado;
paciente *m* (enfermo *m*) interno
i paziente *m* (malato *m*) ospedalizzato
n klinische patiënt;
opgenomen patiënt
d stationärer Patient *m*;
stationärer Krankenhauspatient *m*;
Stationärer *m*

157 BED PLAN
f lits *mpl* prévus par l'état
e camas *fpl* planificadas
i fabbisogno *m* letti previsto dallo stato
n wettelijk voorzien aantal *n* bedden
d Planbetten *npl*

158 BED PLANNING
f planification *f* des lits
e planificación *f* de camas
i pianificazione *f* dei letti
n bedplanning
d Bettenplanung *f*

159 BED-POPULATION RATE;
BED-POPULATION RATIO
f proportion *f* lits-population
e proporción *f* camas-población
i rapporto *m* popolazione-letti
n verhouding bedden-bevolking
d Verhältnis *n* Betten-Bevölkerung

160 BED-POPULATION RATIO
see: BED POPULATION RATE

161 BED REQUIREMENT;
see: BED NEED

162 BEDRIDDEN PATIENT;
NON-AMBULANT PATIENT
f malade *m* (patient *m*) alité;
malade *m* (patient *m*) couché;
malade *m* (patient *m*) grabataire;
malade *m* (patient *m*) non-ambulant
e paciente *m* (enfermo *m*) encamado;
paciente *m* (enfermo *m*) no-ambulante
i malato *m* obbligato a letto;
malato *m* non in grado di alzarsi
n bedlegerige patiënt;
niet-ambulante patiënt
d bettlägeriger Patient *m* (Kranker *m*);
nicht-ambulanter Patient *m* (Kranker *m*)

163 BED SEPARATION
f séparation *f* de lits
e separación *f* de camas
i separazione *f* dei letti
n bedseparatie
d Bettrennung *f*

164 BED STERILIZING ROOM
see: AIR LOCK

165 BED STORE
f entrepôt *m* de lits
e depósito *m* de camas
i deposito *m* dei letti
n beddenmagazijn *n*;
beddendepot *n*
d Bettendepot *n*

166 BED SURPLUS
f surplus *m* de lits
e sobrante *m* de camas
i surplus *m* di letti
n beddenoverschot *n*
d Bettenüberschuss *m*

167 BED UTILIZATION
f utilisation *f* des lits
e utilización *f* de camas
i utilizzazione *f* dei letti
n beddengebruik *n*
d Bettenausnutzung *f*

168 BIBLIOTHERAPY
f bibliothérapie *f*
e biblioterapia *f*
i biblioterapia *f*
n bibliotherapie
d Bibliotherapie *f*

169 BIOCHEMICAL LABORATORY;
BIOCHEMISTRY LABORATORY
f laboratoire *m* biochimique;
laboratoire *m* de biochimie
e laboratorio *m* bioquímico;
laboratorio *m* de bioquímica
i laboratorio *m* biochimico;
laboratorio *m* di biochimica
n biochemisch laboratorium *n*
d biochemisches Laboratorium *n*;
Laboratorium *n* für Biochemie

170 BIOCHEMIST
f biochimiste *m*
e bioquímico *m*
i biochimico *m*
n biochemicus
d Biochemiker *m*

171 BIOCHEMISTRY
f biochimie *f*
e bioquímica *f*
i biochimica *f*;
chimica *f* biologica
n biochemie
d Biochemie *f*

172 BIOCHEMISTRY LABORATORY
see: BIOCHEMICAL LABORATORY

173 BIOLOGICAL CLINICAL LABORATORY
f laboratoire *m* de biologie clinique
e laboratorio *m* de biología clínica
i laboratorio *m* di biologia clinica
n laboratorium *n* voor klinische biologie
d Laboratorium *n* für klinische Biologie

174 BIOLOGICAL LABORATORY;
BIOLOGY LABORATORY
f laboratoire *m* biologique;
laboratoire *m* de biologie
e laboratorio *m* biológico;
laboratorio *m* de biología
i laboratorio *m* di analisi biologiche
n biologisch laboratorium *n*
d biologisches Laboratorium *n*;
Laboratorium *n* für Biologie

175 BIOLOGY LABORATORY
see: BIOLOGICAL LABORATORY

176 BIOMEDICAL RESEARCH
f recherche *f* biomédicale
e investigación *f* biomédica
i ricerca *f* medico-biologica
n biomedisch onderzoek *n*
d biomedizinische Forschung *f*

177 BIOPSY APPARATUS
f appareils *mpl* de biopsie
e aparatos *mpl* de biopsia
i apparecchi *mpl* per la biopsia

n biopsie-apparatuur
d Biopsiegeräte *npl*

178 BIOSTATISTICIAN
f biostatisticien *m*
e bioestadista *m*
i medico *m* che si occupa di statistica sanitaria
n biostatisticus
d Biostatistiker *m*

179 BIOSTATISTICS
f biostatistique *f*
e bioestadística *f*
i statistica *f* medica e sanitaria
n biostatistiek
d Biostatistik *f*

180 BIRTH CONTROL
f contrôle *m* des naissances
e control *m* de natalidades
i controllo *m* delle nascite
n geboortenregeling
d Geburtenregelung *f*

181 BIRTH-RATE;
NATALITY
f natalité *f*
e cifra *f* natalicia;
natalidad *f*
i natalità *f*
n geboortencijfer *n*;
nataliteit
d Geburtenziffer *f*

182 BLOOD BANK
f banque *f* de sang
e banco *m* de sangre
i banca *f* del sangue
n bloedbank
d Blutbank *f*

183 BLOOD DEPOT
f dépôt *m* de sang
e depósito *m* de sangre
i deposito *m* del sangue
n bloeddepot *n*
d Blutdepot *n*

184 BLOOD DONOR
f donneur *m* de sang
e dador *m* de sangre
i donatore *m* di sangue
n bloeddonor
d Blutspender *m*

185 BLOOD EXAMINATION;
BLOOD TEST
f analyse *f* du sang;
analyse *f* sanguine;
examen *m* du sang;
examen *m* sanguin
e análisis *m/f* de sangre
i analisi *f* del sangue;
esame *m* del sangue
n bloedonderzoek *n*
d Blutuntersuchung *f*;
Blutprobe *f*

186 BLOOD GROUP
f groupe *m* sanguin
e grupo *m* hemático;
grupo *m* sanguíneo
i gruppo *m* sanguigno
n bloedgroep
d Blutgruppe *f*

187 BLOOD GROUPING
f détermination *f* du groupe sanguin
e determinación *f* del grupo hemático (sanguíneo)
i determinazione *f* del gruppo sanguigno
n bloedgroepbepaling
d Blutgruppenbestimmung *f*

188 BLOOD LANCET
f vaccinostyle *m*
e sangradera *f*
i vaccinostilo *m*
n bloedlancet *n*
d Blutlanzette *f*

189 BLOOD TEST
see: BLOOD EXAMINATION

190 BLOOD TRANSFUSION
f transfusion *f* sanguine;
transfusion *f* de sang
e transfusión *f* de sangre
i trasfusione *f* di sangue
n bloedtransfusie
d Bluttransfusion *f*

191 BLOOD TRANSFUSION CENTRE (CENTER)
f centre *m* de transfusion sanguine
e centro *m* de transfusión de sangre
i centro *m* trasfusionale
n bloedtranfusiecentrum *n*
d Bluttransfusionszentrum *n*;
Blutspendezentrum *n*

192 BLOOD TRANSFUSION DEPARTMENT
f service *m* (département *m*) de transfusion sanguine
e servicio *m* (departamento *m*) de transfusión de sangre
i servizio *m* trasfusionale
n bloedtransfusie-afdeling
d Bluttransfusionsabteilung *f*;
Blutspendeabteilung *f*

193 BLOOD TRANSFUSION SERVICE
f service *m* de transfusion sanguine
e servicio *m* de transfusión de sangre
i servizio *m* di trasfusione
n bloedtransfusiedienst
d Bluttransfusionsdienst *m*;
Blutspendedienst *m*

194 BLOOD TRANSPORT
f transport *m* de sang
e transporte *m* de sangre
i trasporto *m* di sangue
n bloedtransport *n*
d Bluttransport *m*

195 BLOOD VESSEL BANK
f banque *f* de vaisseaux sanguins
e banco *m* de vasos de sangre
i banca *f* dei vasi sanguigni
n bloedvatenbank
d Blutgefässbank *f*

196 BODILY CARE
f soins *mpl* corporels
e cuidado *m* corporal
i cure *fpl* corporali

n lichaamsverzorging
d Körperpflege *f*

197 BONE BANK
f banque *f* d'os
e banco *m* de huesos
i banca *f* delle ossa
n botbank
d Knochenbank *f*

198 BRAIN BANK
f banque *f* de cerveaux
e banco *m* de sesos
i banca *f* dei cervelli
n hersenbank
d Gehirnbank *f*

199 BURNS CENTRE (CENTER)
f centre *m* des brûlés
e centro *m* de quemados
i centro *m* ustionati
n centrum *n* voor patiënten met (zware) brandwonden; brandwondencentrum *n*
d Zentrum *n* für Brandverletzte; Schwerverbranntenzentrum *n*; Verbranntenzentrum *n*

200 BURNS DEPARTMENT
f service *m* (département *m*) des brûlés
e servicio *m* (departamento *m*) de quemados
i servizio *m* ustionati
n afdeling voor patiënten met (zware) brandwonden
d Abteilung *f* für Brandverletzte; Schwerverbranntenabteilung *f*; Verbranntenabteilung *f*

201 BURNS UNIT
f unité *f* des brûlés
e unidad *f* de quemados
i unità *f* ustionati
n eenheid voor patiënten met (zware) brandwonden
d Station *f* für Verbrennungspatienten; Schwerverbranntenstation *f*; Verbranntenstation *f*

C

202 CADAVER;
CORPSE;
DEAD BODY
f cadavre *m*
e cadáver *m*
i cadavere *m*
n lijk *n*
d Leiche *f*

203 CANCER CARE
f soins *mpl* aux cancéreux
e cuidado *m* (atención *f*) de los cancerosos;
asistencia *f* a los cancerosos
i trattamento *m* dei malati di cancro
n zorg voor kankerpatiënten
d Pflege *f* von Krebspatienten

204 CANCER CENTRE (CENTER)
see: ANTI-CANCER CENTRE (CENTER)

205 CANCER CLINIC
f clinique *f* de cancérologie;
clinique *f* du cancer
e clínica *f* para cáncer;
clínica *f* para cancerológicas
i clinica *f* oncologica;
clinica *f* cancerologica
n kankerkliniek
d Krebsklinik *f*

206 CANCER DEPARTMENT
f service *m* (département *m*) anticancéreux;
service *m* (département *m*) de cancérologie;
service *m* (département *m*) du cancer
e servicio *m* (departamento *m*) para cáncer;
servicio *m* (departamento *m*) para cancerológicas
i divisione *f* di oncologia
n kankerafdeling
d Krebsabteilung *f*

207 CANCER HOSPITAL
f hôpital *m* de cancérologie;
hôpital *m* du cancer
e hospital *m* para cáncer;
hospital *m* para cancerológicas
i ospedale *m* oncologico;
ospedale *m* cancerologico
n kankerziekenhuis *n*
d Krebskrankenhaus *n*

208 CARDIAC CARE
f soins *mpl* cardiologiques
e cuidado *m* cardíaco;
atención *f* cardíaca
i cure *fpl* cardiologiche
n zorg voor hartpatiënten
d Pflege *f* Herzkranker

209 CARDIAC CLINIC;
CARDIOLOGY CLINIC
f clinique *f* cardiologique;
clinique *f* de cardiologie
e clínica *f* cardiológica;
clínica *f* de cardiología
i clinica *f* cardiologica
n hartkliniek;
cardiologische kliniek
d Herzklinik *f*

210 CARDIAC DEPARTMENT;
CARDIOLOGY DEPARTMENT
f service *m* (département *m*) cardiologique;
service *m* (département *m*) de cardiologie
e servicio *m* (departamento *m*) cardiológico;
servicio *m* (departamento *m*) de cardiología
i servizio *m* di cardiologia
n hartafdeling;
cardiologische afdeling
d Herzabteilung *f*

211 CARDIAC HOSPITAL;
CARDIOLOGY HOSPITAL
f hôpital *m* cardiologique;
hôpital *m* de cardiologie
e hospital *m* cardiológico;
hospital *m* de cardiología
i ospedale *m* cardiologico
n hartziekenhuis *n*;
cardiologisch ziekenhuis *n*
d Krankenhaus *n* für Herzkrankheiten

212 CARDIAC PATIENT
f malade *m* (patient *m*) cardiaque;
cardiaque *m*;
cardiac *m*
e paciente *m* (enfermo *m*) cardíaco
i cardiopatico *m*
n hartpatiënt
d Herzkranker *m*

213 CARDIAC REANIMATION;
CARDIAC RESUSCITATION
f réanimation *f* cardiaque
e reanimación *f* cardíaca;
resucitación *f* cardíaca
i rianimazione *f* cardiaca
n hartreanimatie
d Herzreanimation *f*

214 CARDIAC RESUSCITATION
see: CARDIAC REANIMATION

215 CARDIAC UNIT;
CARDIOLOGY UNIT
f unité *f* cardiologique;
unité *f* de cardiologie
e unidad *f* cardiológica;
unidad *f* de cardiología
i unità *f* di cardiologia
n harteenheid;
cardiologische eenheid
d Herzstation *f*

216 CARDIOGRAPH
f cardiographe *m*
e cardiógrafo *m*
i cardiografo *m*
n cardiograaf
d Kardiograph *m*

217 CARDIOLOGIST
f cardiologue *m*
e cardiólogo *m*
i cardiologo *m*
n cardioloog
d Kardiologe *m*

218 CARDIOLOGY
f cardiologie *f*
e cardiología *f*
i cardiologia *f*
n cardiologie
d Kardiologie *f*

219 CARDIOLOGY CENTRE (CENTER);
HEART CENTRE (CENTER)
f centre *m* cardiologique;
centre *m* de cardiologie
e centro *m* cardiológico;
centro *m* de cardiología
i centro *m* cardiologico
n hartcentrum *n*
d Herzzentrum *n*

220 CARDIOLOGY CLINIC
see: CARDIAC CLINIC

221 CARDIOLOGY DEPARTMENT
see: CARDIAC DEPARTMENT

222 CARDIOLOGY HOSPITAL
see: CARDIAC HOSPITAL

223 CARDIOLOGY UNIT
see: CARDIAC UNIT

224 CARDIOVASCULAR DISEASE
f maladie *f* cardio-vasculaire
e enfermedad *f* cardiovascular
i malattia *f* cardio-vascolare
n hart- en vaatziekte
d Herz- und Kreislaufkrankheit *f*

225 CARDIOVASCULAR LABORATORY
f laboratoire *m* cardio-vasculaire
e laboratorio *m* cardiovascular
i laboratorio *m* cardio-vascolare
n cardio-vasculair laboratorium *n*
d Herz- und Kreislauflaboratorium *n*

226 CARDIOVASCULAR NURSING
f soins *mpl* infirmiers cardio-vasculaires
e cuidado *m* enfermero cardiovascular
i cure *fpl* infermieristiche cardio-vascolari
n cardio-vasculaire verpleging
d Herz- und Kreislaufpflege *f*

227 CARDIOVASCULAR OPERATING ROOM;
CARDIOVASCULAR OPERATING THEATRE;
CARDIOVASCULAR OPERATIONS ROOM
f salle *f* d'opérations cardio-vasculaires;
salle *f* opératoire cardio-vasculaire
e sala *f* operatoria cardiovascular;
sala *f* de operaciones cardiovasculares
i sala *f* operatoria cardio-vascolare;
sala *f* d'operazioni cardio-vascolari
n cardio-vasculaire operatiekamer
d Herz- und Kreislaufoperationsraum *m*;
Herz- und Kreislaufoperationssaal *m*

228 CARDIOVASCULAR OPERATING THEATRE
see: CARDIOVASCULAR OPERATING ROOM

229 CARDIOVASCULAR OPERATIONS ROOM
see: CARDIOVASCULAR OPERATING ROOM

230 CARE OF ALCOHOLICS
f soins *mpl* aux alcooliques
e cuidado *m* (atención *f*) de los alcohólicos;
asistencia *f* a los alcohólicos
i trattamento *m* degli alcolizzati
n zorg voor alcoholverslaafden
d Pflege *f* von Alkoholikern

231 CARE OF OLD PEOPLE;
CARE OF THE AGED;
OLD PEOPLE CARE
f soins *mpl* aux personnes âgées
e cuidado *m* (atención *f*) de los ancianos;
asistencia *f* a los ancianos
i cura *f* delle persone anziane;
assistenza *f* alle persone anziane
n bejaardenzorg
d Altenversorgung *f*;
Altenfürsorge *f*

232 CARE OF THE AGED
see: CARE OF OLD PEOPLE

233 CARE OF THE FEEBLE-MINDED;
CARE OF THE MENTALLY DEFECTIVE;
CARE OF THE MENTALLY DEFICIENT;
CARE OF THE MENTALLY DISABLED;
CARE OF THE MENTALLY HANDICAPPED;
CARE OF THE MENTALLY RETARDED;
CARE OF THE MENTALLY SUBNORMAL
f soins *mpl* aux débiles mentaux;
soins *mpl* aux déficients mentaux;
soins *mpl* aux handicapés mentaux;
soins *mpl* aux retardés mentaux
e cuidado *m* (atención *f*) de los débiles mentales;
cuidado *m* (atención *f*) de los atrasados mentales;
cuidado *m* (atención *f*) de los retardados mentales
i cura *f* dei deficienti mentali;
cura *f* degli handicappati mentali
n zwakzinnigenzorg;
zorg voor geestelijk gehandicapten
d Pflege *f* Schwachsinniger;
Pflege *f* Geistesschwacher;
Pflege *f* Geistesbehinderter;
Pflege *f* geistig Behinderter;
Pflege *f* geistig Zurückgebliebener

234 CARE OF THE MENTALLY DEFECTIVE
see: CARE OF THE FEEBLE-MINDED

235 CARE OF THE MENTALLY DEFICIENT
see: CARE OF THE FEEBLE-MINDED

236 CARE OF THE MENTALLY DISABLED
see: CARE OF THE FEEBLE-MINDED

237 CARE OF THE MENTALLY DISEASED;
CARE OF THE MENTALLY ILL

f soins *mpl* aux malades (patients) mentaux
e cuidado *m* (atención *f*) de los pacientes (enfermos) mentales;
asistencia *f* a los pacientes (enfermos) mentales
i cure *fpl* dei malati mentali
n zorg voor psychisch zieken
d Pflege *f* psychisch Kranker;
Pflege *f* Geisteskranker

238 CARE OF THE MENTALLY HANDICAPPED
see: CARE OF THE FEEBLE-MINDED

239 CARE OF THE MENTALLY ILL
see: CARE OF THE MENTALLY DISEASED

240 CARE OF THE MENTALLY RETARDED
see: CARE OF THE FEEBLE-MINDED

241 CARE OF THE MENTALLY SUBNORMAL
see: CARE OF THE FEEBLE-MINDED

242 CASUALTY DEPARTMENT
see: ACCIDENT DEPARTMENT

243 CASUALTY SERVICES
see: ACCIDENT SERVICES

244 CASUALTY TREATMENT
see: ACCIDENT TREATMENT

245 CATHETER
f sonde *f*
e catéter *m*;
sonda *f*
i sonda *f*
n catheter
d Katheter *m*

246 CAUSE OF DISEASE
f cause *f* de maladie
e causa *f* de enfermedad
i causa *f* di malattia
n ziekte-oorzaak
d Krankheitsursache *f*

247 CENTRAL ADMISSION
f admission *f* centrale
e admisión *f* central
i accettazione *f* centrale
n centrale opname
d Zentralaufnahme *f*

248 CENTRAL ADMISSION DEPARTMENT
f service *m* (département *m*) central des admissions
e servicio *m* (departamento *m*) central de admisión
i servizio *m* centrale di accettazione
n centrale opname-afdeling
d zentrale Aufnahmeabteilung *f*

249 CENTRAL ARCHIVES;
CENTRAL FILES;
CENTRAL RECORDS
f archives *fpl* centrales
e archivo *m* central
i archivi *mpl* centrali
n centraal archief *n*
d Zentralarchiv *n*

250 CENTRAL BED CLEANING DEPARTMENT
see: BED CLEANING CENTRE (CENTER)

251 CENTRAL BED SUPPLY
see: BED CENTRE (CENTER)

252 CENTRAL DIAGNOSTIC RADIOLOGICAL DEPARTMENT;
CENTRAL DIAGNOSTIC RADIOLOGY DEPARTMENT;
CENTRAL DIAGNOSTIC X-RAY DEPARTMENT
f service *m* (département *m*) central de radiologie diagnostique;
service *m* (département *m*) central de radiodiagnostic
e servicio *m* (departamento *m*) central de radiología de diagnóstico
i servizio *m* centrale di radiodiagnostica
n centrale röntgendiagnose-afdeling
d zentrale diagnostische Röntgenabteilung *f*;
zentrale röntgendiagnostische Abteilung *f*

253 CENTRAL DIAGNOSTIC RADIOLOGY DEPARTMENT
see: CENTRAL DIAGNOSTIC RADIOLOGICAL DEPARTMENT

254 CENTRAL DIAGNOSTIC X-RAY DEPARTMENT
see: CENTRAL DIAGNOSTIC RADIOLOGICAL DEPARTMENT

255 CENTRAL DRESSING ROOM
f salle *f* centrale de pansement
e sala *f* central de vendaje
i sala *f* centrale di medicazione
n centrale verbandkamer
d zentrales Verbandszimmer *n*

256 CENTRAL FILES
see: CENTRAL ARCHIVES

257 CENTRAL HOSPITAL
f hôpital *m* central
e hospital *m* central
i ospedale *m* centrale
n centraal ziekenhuis *n*;
centrumziekenhuis *n*
d Zentralkrankenhaus *n*;
Schwerpunktkrankenhaus *n*

258 CENTRAL KITCHEN
f cuisine *f* centrale
e cocina *f* central
i cucina *f* centrale
n centrale keuken
d zentrale Küche *f*

259 CENTRAL LABORATORY
f laboratoire *m* central
e laboratorio *m* central
i laboratorio *m* centrale
n centraal laboratorium *n*
d Zentrallaboratorium *n*

260 CENTRAL LAUNDRY
f buanderie *f* centrale
e lavadero *m* central
i lavanderia *f* centrale
n centrale wasserij
d Zentralwäscherei *f*

261 CENTRAL PHARMACY
f pharmacie *f* centrale
e farmacia *f* central
i farmacia *f* centrale
n centrale apotheek
d Zentralapotheke *f*

262 CENTRAL RADIOLOGICAL DEPARTMENT;
CENTRAL RADIOLOGY DEPARTMENT;
CENTRAL X-RAY DEPARTMENT
f service *m* (département *m*) central radiologique;
service *m* (département *m*) central de radiologie;
service *m* (département *m*) central de rayons x
e servicio *m* (departamento *m*) central radiológico;
servicio *m* (departamento *m*) central de radiología;
servicio *m*(departamento *m*) central de rayos x
i servizio *m* centrale di radiologia;
servizio *m* centrale dei raggi x
n centrale röntgenafdeling;
centrale radiologische afdeling;
centrale radiologie-afdeling
d zentrale Röntgenabteilung *f*;
zentrale radiologische Abteilung *f*;
zentrale Radiologieabteilung *f*

263 CENTRAL RADIOLOGY DEPARTMENT
see: CENTRAL RADIOLOGICAL DEPARTMENT

264 CENTRAL RECORDS
see: CENTRAL ARCHIVES

265 CENTRAL STERILIZATION
f stérilisation *f* centrale;
stérilisation *f* centralisée
e esterilización *f* central;
esterilización *f* centralizada
i sterilizzazione *f* centrale
n centrale sterilisatie
d Zentralsterilisation *f*;
zentrale Sterilisation *f*

266 CENTRAL STERILIZATION APPARATUS;
CENTRAL STERILIZATION PLANT;
CENTRAL STERILIZING APPARATUS;
CENTRAL STERILIZING PLANT
f appareils *mpl* de stérilisation centrale
e aparatos *mpl* para esterilización centralizada
i apparecchi *mpl* di sterilizzazione centrale
n centrale sterilisatie-apparatuur
d zentrale Sterilisiergeräte *npl*

267 CENTRAL STERILIZATION DEPARTMENT;
CENTRAL STERILIZING DEPARTMENT
f service *m* (département *m*) central de stérilisation
e servicio *m* (departamento *m*) central de esterilización;
central *f* de esterilización
i servizio *m* centrale di sterilizzazione;
centrale *f* di sterilizzazione
n centrale sterilisatie-afdeling
d Zentralsterilisationsabteilung *f*

268 CENTRAL STERILIZATION PLANT
see: CENTRAL STERILIZATION APPARATUS

269 CENTRAL STERILIZING APPARATUS
see: CENTRAL STERILIZATION APPARATUS

270 CENTRAL STERILIZING DEPARTMENT
see: CENTRAL STERILIZATION DEPARTMENT

271 CENTRAL STERILIZING PLANT
see: CENTRAL STERILIZATION APPARATUS

272 CENTRAL SUPPLY
f approvisionnement *m* central
e abastecimiento *m* central
i approviggionamento *m* centrale
n centrale bevoorrading
d Zentralversorgung *f*

273 CENTRAL SUPPLY DEPARTMENT
f service *m* (département *m*) central d'approvisionnement
e servicio *m* (departamento *m*) central de abastecimiento
i servizio *m* centrale d'approviggionamento
n centrale bevoorradingsafdeling
d Zentralversorgungsabteilung *f*

274 CENTRAL X-RAY DEPARTMENT
see: CENTRAL RADIOLOGICAL DEPARTMENT

275 CHANGING ROOM
f box *m* de déshabillage
e cuarto *m* de vestirse
i spogliatoio *m*
n omkleedruimte
d Umkleidekabine *f*

276 CHEMICAL LABORATORY;
CHEMISTRY LABORATORY
f laboratoire *m* chimique;
laboratoire *m* de chimie
e laboratorio *m* químico
i laboratorio *m* chimico
n chemisch laboratorium *n*
d chemisches Laboratorium *n*

277 CHEMISTRY LABORATORY
see: CHEMICAL LABORATORY

278 CHIEF DOCTOR;
CHIEF PHYSICIAN;
HEAD PHYSICIAN;
MEDICAL CHIEF;
MEDICAL SUPERINTENDENT
f médecin-chef *m*;
médecin-chef *m* de service;
chef *m* de clinique
e médico *m* jefe
i primario *m*
n hoofdgeneesheer
d Chefarzt *m*;
leitender Arzt *m*;
Oberarzt *m*

279 CHIEF MEDICAL OFFICER;
MEDICAL DIRECTOR
f directeur *m* médical;
directeur *m* sanitaire;
médecin-directeur *m*
e director *m* médico;
médico-director *m*
i direttore *m* sanitario
n medisch directeur;
directeur-geneesheer
d ärztlicher Direktor *m*

280 CHIEF NURSE;
HEAD NURSE;
SISTER
f infirmière-chef *f*;
infirmière *f* en chef;
surveillante *f*
e enfermera *f* jefe
i infermiera-capo *f*
n hoofdverpleegkundige;
hoofdverplegende;
hoofdverpleegster;
hoofdzuster
d Oberschwester *f*;
Oberkrankenschwester *f*;
Hauptschwester *f*;
Hauptkrankenschwester *f*;
leitende Schwester *f*

281 CHIEF NURSING OFFICER;
DIRECTOR OF NURSING;
DIRECTOR OF NURSING SERVICE
f directrice *f* (supérieure);
infirmière *f* directrice (des soins);
directrice *f* du nursing
e directora *f* de enfermería
i infermiera *f* direttrice generale
n verpleegkundig directrice
d Krankenhausoberin *f*;
Spitaloberin *f*

282 CHIEF PHYSICIAN
see: CHIEF DOCTOR

283 CHILD BED;
MATERNITY BED
f couches *fpl*
e parto *m*;
alumbramiento *m*;
sobreparto *m*
i parto *m*
n kraambed *n*
d Wochenbett *n*;
Kindbett *n*

284 CHILD CARE
f soins *mpl* des enfants;
puériculture *f*
e puericultura *f*
i cura *f* dell'infanzia;
puericultura *f*
n kinderzorg
d Kinderfürsorge *f*

285 CHILD DISEASE;
CHILDREN'S DISEASE
f maladie *f* infantile;
maladie *f* d'enfant
e enfermedad *f* infantil;
enfermedad *f* de niño
i malattia *f* dell'infanzia
n kinderziekte
d Kinderkrankheit *f*

286 CHILD HEALTH SPECIALIST;
CHILDREN'S DOCTOR;
CHILDREN'S SPECIALIST;
PEDIATRICIAN
f médecin *m* infantile;
pédiatre *m*
e médico *m* infantil;
pedíatra *m*
i pediatra *m*
n kinderarts;
jeugdarts
d Kinderarzt *m*

287 CHILD PROTECTION
f protection *f* infantile;
protection *f* de l'enfance
e protección *f* de la infancia;
protección *f* de los niños
i protezione *f* dell'infanzia
n kinderbescherming
d Kinderschutz *m*

288 CHILD PSYCHIATRY
f psychiatrie *f* infantile
e psiquiatría *f* infantil
i psichiatria *f* infantile
n kinderpsychiatrie
d Kinderpsychiatrie *f*

289 CHILDREN'S CLINIC;
PEDIATRIC CLINIC
f clinique *f* d'enfants;
clinique *f* pédiatrique;
clinique *f* de pédiatrie
e clínica *f* para niños;
clínica *f* infantil;
clínica *f* pediátrica;
clínica *f* de pediatría
i clinica *f* pediatrica
n kinderkliniek
d Kinderklinik *f*

290 CHILDREN'S DAY ROOM
f salle *f* de jour pour enfants;
local *m* de jour pour enfants
e sala *f* diurna para niños;
sala *f* de día para niños
i sala *f* di ricreazione per bambini
n kinderdagverblijf *n*
d Kindertagesraum *m*

291 CHILDREN'S DEPARTMENT;
PEDIATRIC DEPARTMENT
f service *m* (département *m*) d'enfants;
service *m* (département *m*) pédiatrique;
service *m* (département *m*) de pédiatrie
e servicio *m* (departamento *m*) para niños;
servicio *m* (departamento *m*) infantil;
servicio *m* (departamento *m*) pediátrico;
servicio *m* (departamento *m*) de pediatría
i divisione *f* di pediatria
n kinderafdeling
d Kinderabteilung *f*;
pädiatrische Abteilung *f*

292 CHILDREN'S DISEASE
see: CHILD DISEASE

293 CHILDREN'S DOCTOR
see: CHILD HEALTH SPECIALIST

294 CHILDREN'S HEALTH CARE;
PEDIATRIC HEALTH CARE
f soins *mpl* sanitaires d'enfants;
soins *mpl* sanitaires pédiatriques;
soins *mpl* de la santé enfantine
e cuidado *m* sanitario de niños;
cuidado *m* sanitario pediátrico;
cuidado *m* de la salud infantil
i assistenza *f* sanitaria dell'infanzia;
assistenza *f* sanitaria pediatrica
n gezondheidszorg voor kinderen;
kindergezondheidszorg
d Kindergesundheitsfürsorge *f*;
Kindergesundheitspflege *f*

295 CHILDREN'S HOSPITAL;
PEDIATRIC HOSPITAL
f hôpital *m* d'enfants;
hôpital *m* pédiatrique;
hôpital *m* de pédiatrie
e hospital *m* para niños;
hospital *m* infantil;
hospital *m* pediátrico;
hospital *m* de pediatría
i ospedale *m* pediatrico
n kinderziekenhuis *n*
d Kinderkrankenhaus *n*;
Kinderspital *n*

296 CHILDREN'S NURSE
f puéricultrice *f*
e puericultora *f*
i puericultrice *f*
n kinderverzorgster
d Kinderschwester *f*;
Kinderpflegerin *f*

297 CHILDREN'S REHABILITATION
f réadaptation *f* d'enfants;
révalidation *f* d'enfants;
réhabilitation *f* d'enfants
e revalidación *f* infantil;
rehabilitación *f* infantil;

readaptación *f* infantil
i rieducazione *f* dell'infanzia
n kinderrevalidatie
d Kinderrehabilitation *f*

298 CHILDREN'S SANATORIUM
f sanatorium *m* d'enfants
e sanatorio *m* para niños
i sanatorio *m* per l'infanzia
n kindersanatorium *n*
d Kindersanatorium *n*

299 CHILDREN'S SPECIALIST
see: CHILD HEALTH SPECIALIST

300 CHILDREN'S UNIT;
PEDIATRIC UNIT
f unité *f* d'enfants;
unité *f* pédiatrique;
unité *f* de pédiatrie
e unidad *f* para niños;
unidad *f* infantil;
unidad *f* pediátrica;
unidad *f* de pediatría
i unità *f* di pediatria
n kindereenheid
d Kinderstation *f*;
pädiatrische Station *f*

301 CHIROPODIST;
PODIATRIST
f pédicure *m*
e giropodista *m*
i chiropodista *m*
n chiropodist;
voetverzorger
d Fusspfleger *m*

302 CHIROPODY;
PODIATRY
f soins *mpl* du pédicure
e giropodía *f*
i chiropodia *f*
n chiropodie;
voetverzorging
d Fusspflege *f*

303 CHOICE OF MEALS
f choix *m* des repas
e elección *f* de comidas
i scelta *f* dei pasti
n maaltijdkeuze
d Wahlessen *n*

304 CHRONIC CARE;
CHRONIC ILLNESS CARE;
CHRONIC PATIENT CARE;
CHRONIC SICK CARE;
LONG STAY (PATIENT) CARE;
LONG TERM (PATIENT) CARE
f soins *mpl* aux chroniques;
soins *mpl* aux malades (patients) chroniques;
soins *mpl* de longue durée
e cuidado *m* (atención *f*) de los pacientes (enfermos) crónicos;
cuidado *m* (atención *f*) a largo plazo;
cuidado *m* (atención *f*) de larga duración
i cura *f* dei malati cronici;
assistenza *f* ai malati cronici;
cura *f* di lunga durata
n zorg voor chronische patiënten;
zorg voor langdurig zieken
d Fürsorge *f* für Chronischkranke
(chronisch Erkrankte, Chroniker, Langzeitkranke, Langfristigkranke);
Siechenpflege *f*;
Langzeitpflege *f*

305 CHRONIC CARE INSTITUTION;
CHRONIC DISEASE (ILLNESS, SICK) HOSPITAL;
HOME FOR LONG STAY PATIENTS;
LONG STAY (CARE) INSTITUTION;
LONG STAY HOSPITAL;
LONG TERM (CARE) INSTITUTION;
LONG TERM HOSPITAL;
NURSING CENTRE (CENTER);
NURSING HOME
f hôpital *m* (institution *f*, établissement *m*) pour malades chroniques;
hôpital *m* de long séjour;
hôpital *m* pour maladies de longue durée;
établissement *m* à long terme;
maison *f* de santé;
établissement *m* de soins
e hospital *m* (institución *f*) para pacientes (enfermos) crónicos;
hospital *m* (institución *f*) de largo plazo;
casa *f* de salud;
establecimiento-enfermería *m*
i ospedale *m* (istituto *m*) per malati cronici e per lungodegenti
n ziekenhuis *n* (inrichting) voor chronische patiënten;
verpleeghuis *n*;
verpleeginrichting
d Krankenhaus *n* (Institution *f*) für Chronischkranke;
Chronikerkrankenhaus *n*;
Langaufenthaltsanstalt *f*;
Langzeitbehandlungsanstalt *f*;
Pflegeheim *n*;
Pflegeanstalt *f*;
Pflegehaus *n*;
Versorgungsheim *n*;
Krankenheim *n*

306 CHRONIC DISEASE (ILLNESS, SICKNESS);
LONG TERM DISEASE (ILLNESS, SICKNESS)
f maladie *f* chronique;
maladie *f* de longue durée
e enfermedad *f* crónica;
enfermedad *f* de largo plazo
i malattia *f* cronica;
malattia *f* di lunga durata
n chronische ziekte;
langdurige ziekte
d chronische Krankheit *f*;
Langzeitkrankheit *f*

307 CHRONIC DISEASE (ILLNESS) FACILITIES;
LONG STAY FACILITIES;
LONG TERM FACILITIES
f services *mpl* pour malades (patients) chroniques
e servicios *mpl* para pacientes (enfermos) crónicos
i servizi *mpl* per malati cronici
n voorzieningen voor chronische patiënten
d Dienste *mpl* für Chronischkranke

308 CHRONIC DISEASE HOSPITAL
see: CHRONIC CARE INSTITUTION

309 CHRONIC ILLNESS
see: CHRONIC DISEASE

310 CHRONIC ILLNESS CARE
see: CHRONIC CARE

311 CHRONIC ILLNESS DEPARTMENT;
CHRONIC SICK DEPARTMENT;
LONG STAY DEPARTMENT;
LONG TERM DEPARTMENT
f service *m* (département *m*) pour malades (patients) chroniques
e servicio *m* (departamento *m*) para pacientes (enfermos) crónicos
i divisione *f* degli ammalati cronici
n afdeling voor chronische patiënten
d Abteilung *f* für Chronischkranke

312 CHRONIC ILLNESS FACILITIES
see: CHRONIC DISEASE FACILITIES

313 CHRONIC ILLNESS HOSPITAL
see: CHRONIC CARE INSTITUTION

314 CHRONIC ILLNESS NURSING;
CHRONIC SICK NURSING;
LONG STAY NURSING;
LONG TERM NURSING
f soins *mpl* infirmiers aux malades (patients) chroniques
e cuidado *m* enfermero de los pacientes (enfermos) crónicos
i assistenza *f* infermieristica agli ammalati cronici
n verpleging van chronische patiënten
d Pflege *f* Chronischkranker

315 CHRONIC ILLNESS UNIT;
CHRONIC SICK UNIT;
LONG STAY UNIT;
LONG TERM UNIT
f unité *f* pour malades (patients) chroniques
e unidad *f* para pacientes (enfermos) crónicos
i unità *f* degli ammalati cronici
n eenheid voor chronische patiënten
d Einheit *f* für Chronischkranke

316 CHRONIC PATIENT;
CHRONIC SICK;
LONG STAY PATIENT;
LONG TERM PATIENT
f malade *m* (patient *m*) chronique;
chronique *m*
e paciente *m* (enfermo *m*) crónico;
paciente *m* (enfermo *m*) de larga enfermedad
i malato *m* cronico
n chronische patiënt;
chronisch zieke;
langdurig zieke
d Chronischkranker *m*;
chronisch Erkrankter *m*;
Chroniker *m*;
Langzeitkranker *m*;
Langfristigkranker *m*

317 CHRONIC PATIENT CARE
see: CHRONIC CARE

318 CHRONIC SICK
see: CHRONIC PATIENT

319 CHRONIC SICK CARE
see: CHRONIC CARE

320 CHRONIC SICK DEPARTMENT
see: CHRONIC ILLNESS DEPARTMENT

321 CHRONIC SICK HOSPITAL
see: CHRONIC CARE INSTITUTION

322 CHRONIC SICKNESS
see: CHRONIC DISEASE

323 CHRONIC SICK NURSING
see: CHRONIC ILLNESS NURSING

324 CHRONIC SICK UNIT
see: CHRONIC ILLNESS UNIT

325 CITY HOSPITAL;
URBAN HOSPITAL
f hôpital *m* urbain
e hospital *m* urbano
i ospedale *m* urbano
n stadsziekenhuis *n*;
stedelijk ziekenhuis *n*
d Stadtkrankenhaus *n*;
städtisches Krankenhaus *n*

326 CIVIL MEDICINE
f médecine *f* civile
e medicina *f* civil
i medicina *f* civile
n burgerlijke geneeskunde
d Zivilmedizin *f*

327 CLASSLESS HOSPITAL
f hôpital *m* sans classes
e hospital *m* sin clases
i ospedale *m* senza categorie di paganti
n klassenloos ziekenhuis *n*
d klassenloses Krankenhaus *n*

328 CLINIC
f clinique *f*
e clínica *f*
i clinica *f*
n kliniek
d Klinik *f*

329 CLINICAL APPARATUS
f appareils *mpl* cliniques
e aparatos *mpl* clínicos
i apparecchi *mpl* clinici
n klinische apparatuur
d klinische Geräte *npl*

330 CLINICAL ARCHIVES;
CLINICAL FILES;
CLINICAL RECORDS
f archives *fpl* cliniques
e archivo *m* clínico
i archivi *mpl* clinici
n klinisch archief *n*
d klinisches Archiv *n*

331 CLINICAL BIOCHEMISTRY LABORATORY
f laboratoire *m* de biochimie clinique;
laboratoire *m* de chimie biologique clinique
e laboratorio *m* de bioquímica clínica
i laboratorio *m* di biochimica clinica;
laboratorio *m* di chimica biologica clinica
n laboratorium *n* voor klinische biochemie
d Laboratorium *n* für klinische Biochemie

332 CLINICAL CARE;
INPATIENT CARE
f soins *mpl* cliniques;
soins *mpl* en clinique
e cuidado *m* clínico;
atención *f* clínica
i cure *fpl* cliniche

n klinische zorg
d klinische Fürsorge *f*;
stationäre Fürsorge *f*

333 CLINICAL CARE UNIT
f unité *f* de soins cliniques
e unidad *f* de cuidado clínico
i unità *f* di cure cliniche
n eenheid voor klinische zorg
d Station *f* für klinische Pflege

334 CLINICAL CENTRE (CENTER)
f centre *m* clinique
e centro *m* clínico
i centro *m* clinico
n klinisch centrum *n*
d klinisches Zentrum *n*

335 CLINICAL CHEMIST
f chimiste *m* clinique
e químico *m* clínico
i chimico *m* clinico
n klinisch chemicus
d klinischer Chemiker *m*

336 CLINICAL CHEMISTRY
f chimie *f* clinique
e química *f* clínica
i chimica *f* clinica
n klinische chemie
d klinische Chemie *f*

337 CLINICAL CHEMISTRY LABORATORY
f laboratoire *m* de chimie clinique
e laboratorio *m* clínico-químico
i laboratorio *m* di chimica clinica
n klinisch-chemisch laboratorium *n*
d Laboratorium *n* für klinische Chemie;
klinisch-chemisches Laboratorium *n*

338 CLINICAL DEMONSTRATION ROOM
f salle *f* de présentation clinique
e sala *f* de presentación clínica
i sala *f* di presentazione clinica
n klinische demonstratiezaal
d klinischer Demonstrationsraum *m*

339 CLINICAL FILES
see: CLINICAL ARCHIVES

340 CLINICAL HEALTH CARE;
INPATIENT HEALTH CARE
f soins *mpl* sanitaires cliniques;
soins *mpl* sanitaires en clinique
e cuidado *m* sanitario clínico;
atención *f* sanitaria clínica
i cure *fpl* sanitarie cliniche
n klinische gezondheidszorg
d klinische Gesundheitsfürsorge *f*;
stationäre Gesundheitsfürsorge *f*

341 CLINICAL IMMUNOLOGY LABORATORY
f laboratoire *m* d'immunologie clinique
e laboratorio *m* clínico de inmunología
i laboratorio *m* d'immunologia clinica
n klinisch-immunologisch laboratorium *n*
d klinisches immunologisches Laboratorium *n*

342 CLINICAL INVESTIGATION LABORATORY
f laboratoire *m* d'analyses cliniques
e laboratorio *m* de investigación clínica
i laboratorio *m* di analisi cliniche
n klinisch onderzoekslaboratorium *n*
d klinisches Forschungslaboratorium *n*

343 CLINICAL LABORATORY
f laboratoire *m* clinique
e laboratorio *m* clínico
i laboratorio *m* clinico
n klinisch laboratorium *n*
d klinisches Laboratorium *n*

344 CLINICAL MEDICINE
f médecine *f* clinique
e medicina *f* clínica
i medicina *f* clinica
n klinische geneeskunde
d klinische Medizin *f*

345 CLINICAL MENTAL CARE;
CLINICAL MENTAL HEALTH CARE;
CLINICAL PSYCHIATRIC CARE
f soins *mpl* psychiatriques cliniques;
soins *mpl* mentaux cliniques
e cuidado *m* psiquiátrico clínico;
cuidado *m* mental clínico;
atención *f* (asistencia *f*) psiquiátrica clínica;
atención (asistencia *f*) mental clínica
i cure *fpl* psichiatriche cliniche
n klinische geestelijke gezondheidszorg;
klinische psychiatrische zorg
d klinische psychiatrische Fürsorge *f*;
klinische psychiatrische Versorgung *f*

346 CLINICAL MENTAL HEALTH CARE
see: CLINICAL MENTAL CARE

347 CLINICAL NURSE
f infirmière *f* clinique
e enfermera *f* clínica
i infermiera *f* clinica
n klinische verpleegster
d klinische Pflegerin *f*

348 CLINICAL PATHOLOGY
f biologie *f* médicale
e patología *f* clínica
i biologia *f* medica
n klinische pathologie
d klinische Pathologie *f*

349 CLINICAL PHARMACY
f pharmacie *f* clinique
e farmacia *f* clínica
i farmacia *f* clinica
n klinische apotheek
d klinische Apotheke *f*

350 CLINICAL PICTURE;
SYNDROME
f syndrome *m*
e cuadro *m* patológico;
cuadro *m* morboso;
síndrome *m*
i sindrome *f*
n ziektebeeld *n*
d Krankheitsbild *n*

351 CLINICAL PSYCHIATRIC CARE
see: CLINICAL MENTAL CARE

352 CLINICAL PSYCHIATRY
f psychiatrie *f* clinique
e psiquiatría *f* clínica

i psichiatria *f* clinica
n klinische psychiatrie
d klinische Psychiatrie *f*

353 CLINICAL PSYCHOLOGIST
f psychologue *m* clinique
e psicólogo *m* clínico
i psicologo *m* clinico
n klinisch psycholoog
d klinischer Psychologe *m*

354 CLINICAL PSYCHOLOGY
f psychologie *f* clinique
e psicología *f* clínica
i psicologia *f* clinica
n klinische psychologie
d klinische Psychologie *f*

355 CLINICAL RADIOLOGY
f radiologie *f* clinique
e radiología *f* clínica
i radiologia *f* clinica
n klinische radiologie
d klinische Radiologie *f*

356 CLINICAL RECORDS
see: CLINICAL ARCHIVES

357 CLINICAL RESEARCH
f recherche *f* clinique
e investigación *f* clínica
i ricerca *f* clinica
n klinisch onderzoek *n*
d klinische Forschung *f*

358 CLINICAL SERVICES
f services *mpl* cliniques
e servicios *mpl* clínicos
i servizi *mpl* clinici
n klinische diensten
d klinische Dienste *mpl*

359 CLINICAL SPECIALIST
f spécialiste *m* clinique
e especialista *m* clínico
i specialista *m* clinico
n klinisch specialist
d klinischer Facharzt *m*;
klinischer Spezialarzt *m*

360 CLINICAL TREATMENT;
INPATIENT TREATMENT
f traitement *m* clinique;
traitement *m* en clinique
e tratamiento *m* clínico
i trattamento *m* clinico
n klinische behandeling
d klinische Behandlung *f*;
stationäre Behandlung *f*

361 CLINICIAN
f clinicien *m*
e clínico *m*
i clinico *m*
n klinicus;
clinist
d Kliniker *m*

362 COAGULATION LABORATORY
f laboratoire *m* de coagulation
e laboratorio *m* de coagulación
i laboratorio *m* di coagulazione
n stollingslaboratorium *n*
d Koagulationslaboratorium *n*

363 COBALT THERAPY
f cobalthérapie *f*
e cobaltoterapia *f*
i cobaltoterapia *f*
n cobalttherapie
d Kobalttherapie *f*

364 COLD KITCHEN
f cuisine *f* froide
e cocina *f* fría
i cucina *f* fredda
n koude keuken
d kalte Küche *f*

365 COMMON ROOM
f salle *f* commune
e sala *f* general
i sala *f* comune
n meerbedskamer
d Mehrbettzimmer *n*

366 COMMUNICABLE DISEASE;
CONTAGIOUS DISEASE;
INFECTIOUS DISEASE
f maladie *f* contagieuse;
maladie *f* infectieuse;
maladie *f* transmissible
e enfermedad *f* contagiosa;
enfermedad *f* infecciosa;
enfermedad *f* infectiva
i malattia *f* infettiva
n besmettelijke ziekte
d ansteckende Krankheit *f*;
übertragbare Krankheit *f*;
Infektionskrankheit *f*

367 COMMUNICABLE DISEASE CARE;
CONTAGIOUS DISEASE CARE;
INFECTIOUS DISEASE CARE
f soins *mpl* des maladies contagieuses (infectieuses)
e cuidado *m* (atención *f*) de las enfermedades contagiosas (infecciosas)
i cura *f* delle malattie infettive
n zorg voor besmettelijke ziekten
d Infektionsversorgung *f*

368 COMMUNICABLE DISEASE CLINIC;
CONTAGIOUS DISEASE CLINIC;
INFECTIOUS DISEASE CLINIC
f clinique *f* des maladies contagieuses (infectieuses)
e clínica *f* de enfermedades contagiosas (infecciosas)
i clinica *f* per le malattie infettive
n kliniek voor besmettelijke ziekten
d Infektionsklinik *f*

369 COMMUNICABLE DISEASE CONTROL;
CONTAGIOUS DISEASE CONTROL;
INFECTIOUS DISEASE CONTROL
f lutte *f* contre les maladies contagieuses (infectieuses)
e lucha *f* contra enfermedades contagiosas (infecciosas)
i lotta *f* contro le malattie infettive
n besmettelijke ziektenbestrijding;
bestrijding van besmettelijke ziekten
d Bekämpfung *f* von ansteckenden Krankheiten

370 COMMUNICABLE DISEASE DEPARTMENT;
CONTAGIOUS DISEASE DEPARTMENT;
INFECTIOUS DISEASE DEPARTMENT
f service *m* (département *m*) des maladies contagieuses (infectieuses)

e servicio *m* (departamento *m*) de enfermedades contagiosas (infecciosas)
i divisione *f* per le malattie infettive
n afdeling voor besmettelijke ziekten
d Infektionsabteilung *f*

371 COMMUNICABLE DISEASE HOSPITAL;
CONTAGIOUS DISEASE HOSPITAL;
INFECTIOUS DISEASE HOSPITAL
f hôpital *m* des maladies contagieuses (infectieuses)
e hospital *m* de enfermedades contagiosas (infecciosas)
i ospedale *m* per le malattie infettive
n ziekenhuis *n* voor besmettelijke ziekten
d Infektionskrankenhaus *n*

372 COMMUNICABLE DISEASE NURSING;
CONTAGIOUS DISEASE NURSING;
INFECTIOUS DISEASE NURSING
f soins *mpl* infirmiers aux infectieux
e enfermería *f* de las enfermedades contagiosas (infecciosas)
i cure *fpl* infermieristiche dei contagiosi
n verpleging van besmettelijke ziekten
d Infektionspflege *f*

373 COMMUNICABLE DISEASE UNIT;
CONTAGIOUS DISEASE UNIT;
INFECTIOUS DISEASE UNIT
f unité *f* des maladies contagieuses (infectieuses)
e unidad *f* de enfermedades contagiosas (infecciosas)
i unità *f* per le malattie infettive
n eenheid voor besmettelijke ziekten
d Infektions(pflege)station *f*

374 COMMUNICABLE PATIENT;
CONTAGIOUS PATIENT;
INFECTIOUS PATIENT
f malade *m* (patient *m*) infectieux
e paciente *m* (enfermo *m*) contagioso
i malato *m* infettivo;
malato *m* contagioso
n besmettelijke patiënt
d infektiöser Patient *m* (Kranker *m*)

375 COMPULSORY ADMISSION
f admission *f* obligée
e admisión *f* obligada
i ricovero *m* obbligato
n gedwongen opname
d Zwangaufnahme *f*

376 COMPULSORY HEALTH CARE INSURANCE;
COMPULSORY HEALTH INSURANCE;
OBLIGATORY HEALTH CARE INSURANCE;
OBLIGATORY HEALTH INSURANCE
f assurance *f* maladie obligatoire
e seguro *m* de salud obligatorio;
seguro *m* de enfermedad obligatorio
i assicurazione *f* malattia obbligatoria;
assicurazione *f* contro le malattie obbligatoria
n verplichte ziekte(kosten)verzekering
d Pflichtkrankenversicherung *f*

377 COMPULSORY HEALTH INSURANCE
see: COMPULSORY HEALTH CARE INSURANCE

378 COMPULSORY INSURED PERSON
f assuré *m* obligatoire
e asegurado *m* obligatorio
i assicurato *m* d'obbligo
n verplicht verzekerde
d Pflichtversicherter *m*

379 COMPULSORY VACCINATION
f vaccination *f* obligatoire
e vacunación *f* obligatoria
i vaccinazione *f* obbligatoria
n vaccinatiedwang;
verplichte vaccinatie
d Impfpflicht *f*;
Impfzwang *m*

380 CONNECTIVE TISSUE DISEASE
f maladie *f* de tissu conjonctif
e enfermedad *f* de tejido celular
i malattia *f* del tessuto connettivo
n bindweefselziekte
d Bindegewebekrankheit *f*

381 CONSULTANT;
MEDICAL SPECIALIST;
REGISTRAR;
SPECIALIST
f médecin *m* spécialiste;
spécialiste *m*
e médico *m* especialista;
especialista *m* médico;
especialista *m*
i medico *m* specialista;
specialista *m*
n medisch specialist;
specialist
d Facharzt *m*;
Spezialarzt *m*

382 CONSULTANT PHYSICIAN
f médecin-consultant *m*
e médico *m* consultante
i medico *m* consulente
n adviserend arts
d Konsiliararzt *m*

383 CONSULTATION
f consultation *f*
e consulta *f*
i consulto *m*
n consultatie;
consult *n*
d Konsultation *f*

384 CONSULTATION HOUR;
CONSULTING HOUR
f heure *f* de consultation
e hora *f* de consulta
i ora *f* di consulto
n spreekuur *n*
d Sprechstunde *f*

385 CONSULTATION ROOM;
CONSULTING ROOM
f salle *f* de consultation;
cabinet *m* de consultation
e sala *f* de consultas
i sala *f* di visita medica;
ambulatorio *m* medico
n spreekkamer
d Sprechzimmer *n*

386 CONSULTING HOUR
see: CONSULTATION HOUR

387 CONSULTING ROOM
see: CONSULTATION ROOM

388 CONTAGIOUS DISEASE
see: COMMUNICABLE DISEASE

389 CONTAGIOUS DISEASE CARE
see: COMMUNICABLE DISEASE CARE

390 CONTAGIOUS DISEASE CLINIC
see: COMMUNICABLE DISEASE CLINIC

391 CONTAGIOUS DISEASE CONTROL
see: COMMUNICABLE DISEASE CONTROL

392 CONTAGIOUS DISEASE DEPARTMENT
see: COMMUNICABLE DISEASE DEPARTMENT

393 CONTAGIOUS DISEASE HOSPITAL
see: COMMUNICABLE DISEASE HOSPITAL

394 CONTAGIOUS DISEASE NURSING
see: COMMUNICABLE DISEASE NURSING

395 CONTAGIOUS DISEASE UNIT
see: COMMUNICABLE DISEASE UNIT

396 CONTAGIOUS PATIENT
see: COMMUNICABLE PATIENT

397 CONTINUINTY OF CARE
f continuité *f* des soins
e continuidad *f* del cuidado
i continuità *f* delle cure
n continuïteit van de zorg
d Kontinuität *f* der Pflege

398 CONTRIBUTION TO A HEALTH INSURANCE FUND
f cotisation *f* à une caisse d'assurance-maladie
e cuota *f* de una caja de enfermedad
i contributi *mpl* versati ad una cassa mutua
n ziekenfondspremie
d Krankenkassenbeitrag *m*

399 CONVALESCENT CARE
f soins *mpl* aux convalescents
e cuidado *m* (atención *f*) convaleciente
i cura *f* dei convalescenti
n zorg voor herstellenden
d Pflege *f* von Rekonvaleszenten

400 CONVALESCENT DEPARTMENT
f service *m* (département *m*) des convalescents
e servicio *m* (departamento *m*) de convalecencia
i divisione *f* per convalescenti
n afdeling voor herstellenden
d Abteilung *f* für Rekonvaleszenten

401 CONVALESCENT HOME;
CONVALESCENT HOSPITAL
f maison *f* de convalescence;
centre *m* de convalescence
e casa *f* de convalecencia;
hogar *m* de convalecencia
i ospedale *m* per convalescenti
n herstellingsoord *n*;
ziekenhuis *n* voor herstellenden
d Erholungsheim *n*;
Nachsorgekrankenhaus *n*

402 CONVALESCENT HOSPITAL
see: CONVALESCENT HOME

403 CONVALESCENT PATIENT;
RECOVERING PATIENT
f malade *m* (patient *m*) convalescent
e paciente *m* (enfermo *m*) convaleciente
i malato *m* convalescente
n herstellende patiënt
d Rekonvaleszent *m*;
genesender Patient *m* (Kranker *m*)

404 CONVALESCENT UNIT
f unité *f* des convalescents
e unidad *f* de convalecencia
i unità *f* per convalescenti
n eenheid voor herstellenden
d Station *f* für Rekonvaleszenten

405 COPROLOGICAL LABORATORY;
EXCRETA LABORATORY
f laboratoire *m* coprologique
e laboratorio *m* coprológico
i laboratorio *m* coprologico
n faecaliënlaboratorium *n*
d Laboratorium *n* für Koprologie

406 CORONARY CARE
f soins *mpl* aux coronariens
e cuidado *m* coronario;
atención *f* (asistencia *f*) coronaria
i cure *fpl* coronarie
n coronaire zorg
d Pflege *f* Koronarkranker

407 CORONARY CARE UNIT
f unité *f* de soins aux coronariens
e unidad *f* de cuidado coronario;
unidad *f* coronaria
i unità *f* di cure coronarie
n hartbewakingseenheid
d Station *f* für Koronarkranke

408 CORONARY PATIENT
f coronarien *m*
e paciente *m* (enfermo *m*) coronario
i coronarico *m*
n coronaire patiënt
d Koronarkranker *m*

409 CORPSE
see: CADAVER

410 COST OF A STAY
f coût *m* de séjour
e gastos *mpl* de la estancia
i costo *m* del soggiorno
n verblijfskosten
d Aufenthaltskosten *pl*

411 COST OF HOSPITAL CARE;
COST OF HOSPITALIZATION;
COST OF INPATIENT CARE;
HOSPITAL CARE COST;
HOSPITAL COST;
HOSPITALIZATION COST
f coût *m* de l'hospitalisation;
frais *mpl* d'hospitalisation;
frais *mpl* hospitaliers;
frais *mpl* d'hôpital;
prix *m* de revient
e gastos *mpl* de hospitalización;
gastos *mpl* hospitalarios;
gastos *mpl* de hospital

i costo *m* della degenza
n kosten van ziekenhuisverpleging;
verpleegkosten
d Krankenhauskosten *pl*

412 COST OF HOSPITALIZATION
see: COST OF HOSPITAL CARE

413 COST OF ILLNESS
f risque *m* maladie
e gastos *mpl* de enfermedad
i costi *mpl* di malattia
n ziektekosten
d Krankheitskosten *pl*

414 COST OF INPATIENT CARE
see: COST OF HOSPITAL CARE

415 COST PER BED
f coût *m* par lit
e gastos *mpl* por cama
i costo *m* per ciascun letto
n kosten per bed
d Kosten *pl* pro Krankenbett

416 COST PER DAY;
COST PER PATIENT DAY;
DAILY CHARGE;
DAILY COST;
DAILY HOSPITAL CHARGE;
DAILY HOSPITAL COST;
DAILY RATE;
DAY CHARGE;
DAY COST;
DAY RATE
f coût *m* de la (par) journée de malade;
coût *m* de la (par) journée d'hospitalisation;
coût *m* des soins par jour;
prix *m* de (la) journée
e costo *m* por paciente-día;
costo *m* del día de estancia;
precio *m* de (por) la jornada;
precio *m* de día
i costo *m* di una giornata di degenza
n kosten per verpleegdag;
verpleegprijs per dag;
verpleegdagprijs;
dagverpleegprijs;
dagligprijs
d Tages(pflege)satz *m*

417 COST PER PATIENT DAY
see: COST PER DAY

418 COT;
HOSPITAL BED
f lit *m* hospitalier;
lit *m* d'hôpital
e cama *f* hospitalaria;
cama *f* de hospital
i letto *m* d'ospedale
n ziekenhuisbed *n*
d Krankenhausbett *n*

419 COTTAGE HOSPITAL;
RURAL HOSPITAL
f hôpital *m* rural
e hospital *m* rural
i ospedale *m* rurale
n plattelandsziekenhuis *n*
d Landkrankenhaus *n*;
Landspital *n*

420 COURSE OF DISEASE
f marche *f*;
processus *m*;
évolution *f* de la maladie
e proceso *m* de una enfermedad
i evoluzione *f* della malattia
n ziekteverloop *n*;
ziekteproces *n*
d Krankheitsverlauf *m*;
Krankheitsprozess *m*

421 CROSS ASSOCIATION;
CROSS SOCIETY;
HOME NURSING ORGANIZATION
f association *f* d'une croix
e asociación *f* de una cruz
i associazione *f* di una croce
n kruisvereniging
d Organisation *f* der Hauskrankenpflege

422 CROSS INFECTION
f infection *f* croisée;
hospitalisme *m*
e infección *f* cruzada
i infezione *f* crociata
n kruisinfectie
d Mischinfektion *f*

423 CROSS SOCIETY
see: CROSS ASSOCIATION

424 CULTURE ROOM;
INCUBATION ROOM
f salle *f* d'incubation;
enceinte *f* d'incubation
e sala *f* de incubación
i sala *f* d'incubazione
n broedkamer;
kweekruimte
d Brutkammer *f*

425 CURATIVE CARE
f soins *mpl* curatifs
e cuidado *m* curativo;
atención *f* (asistencia *f*) curativa
i trattamento *m* curativo
n curatieve zorg
d kurative Pflege *f*

426 CURATIVE MEDICINE
f médecine *f* curative
e medicina *f* curativa
i medicina *f* curativa
n curatieve geneeskunde
d kurative Medizin *f*;
Heilmedizin *f*

427 CYSTOSCOPY
f cystoscopie *f*
e cistoscopia *f*
i cistoscopia *f*
n cystoscopie
d Zystoskopie *f*

428 CYSTOSCOPY ROOM
f salle *f* de cystoscopie
e sala *f* de cistoscopia
i sala *f* di cistoscopia
n cystoscopieruimte
d Zystoskopieraum *m*

429 CYTOLOGY
f cytologie *f*
e citología *f*
i citologia *f*
n cytologie
d Zytologie *f*

430 CYTOLOGY UNIT
f unité *f* de cytologie
e unidad *f* de citología
i unità *f* di citologia
n cytologie-eenheid
d Zytologiestation *f*

D

431 DAILY CHARGE
see: COST PER DAY

432 DAILY COST
see: COST PER DAY

433 DAILY HOSPITAL CHARGE
see: COST PER DAY

434 DAILY HOSPITAL COST
see: COST PER DAY

435 DAILY RATE
see: COST PER DAY

436 DANCE THERAPY
f thérapie *f* par la dance
e terapia *f* de danza
i terapia *f* mediante l'impiego della danza
n danstherapie
d Tanztherapie *f*

437 DAY CARE
f soins *mpl* de jour
e cuidado *m* diurno;
atención *f* (asistencia *f*) diurna
i cure *fpl* diurne
n dagverzorging
d Tagesversorgung *f*

438 DAY CARE CENTRE (CENTER);
DAY CENTRE (CENTER)
f centre *m* (médical) de jour
e centro *m* diurno;
centro *m* de cuidado diurno (atención diurna, asistencia diurna);
hogar *m* diurno
i centro *m* medico diurno
n centrum *n* voor dagverpleging
d Tageszentrum *n*;
Tagsüber-Pflegezentrum *n*;
Tagesheim *n*;
Tagesstätte *f*

439 DAY CENTRE (CENTER)
see: DAY CARE CENTRE (CENTER)

440 DAY CHARGE
see: COST PER DAY

441 DAY CLINIC
f clinique *f* de jour
e clínica *f* diurna;
clínica *f* de día
i clinica *f* diurna
n dagkliniek
d Tag(es)klinik *f*

442 DAY COST
see: COST PER DAY

443 DAY HOSPITAL
f hôpital *m* de jour
e hospital *m* diurno;
hospital *m* de día
i ospedale *m* diurno
n dagziekenhuis *n*
d Tag(es)krankenhaus *n*;
Tagesspital *n*

444 DAY HOSPITAL FOR CHILDREN
f hôpital *m* de jour pour enfants
e hospital *m* diurno para niños;
hospital *m* de día para niños
i ospedale *m* pediatrico diurno
n kinderdagziekenhuis *n*
d Kindertageskrankenhaus *n*;
Kindertagesspital *n*

445 DAY HOSPITALIZATION
f hospitalisation *f* de jour
e hospitalización *f* diurna;
hospitalización *f* de día
i ospedalizzazione *f* diurna
n daghospitalisatie
d Tagespflege *f* in einem Krankenhaus

446 DAY NURSING
f soins *mpl* infirmiers de jour
e enfermería *f* diurna;
enfermería *f* de día
i cure *fpl* infermieristiche diurne
n dagverpleging
d Tagespflege *f*

447 DAY OF CARE;
DAY OF TREATMENT;
HOSPITAL DAY;
INPATIENT DAY;
INPATIENT SERVICE DAY;
PATIENT DAY
f journée *f* d'hospitalisation;
journée *f* de soins;
journée *f* de malade
e día-paciente *m*;
día-enfermo *m*;
paciente-día *m*;
día *m* de hospitalización;
día *m* de hospital;
día *m* de estancia
i giornata *f* di ospedalizzazione;
giorno *m* di ospedalizzazione
n verpleegdag
d Pflegetag *m*;
Krankenpflegetag *m*;
Krankenhaustag *m*

448 DAY OF TREATMENT
see: DAY OF CARE

449 DAY PATIENT
f malade *m* (patient *m*) de jour
e paciente *m* (enfermo *m*) diurno;
paciente *m* (enfermo *m*) de día
i malato *m* diurno
n dagpatiënt
d Tagespatient *m*;
Tageskranker *m*

450 DAY PSYCHIATRIC TREATMENT
f traitement *m* psychiatrique de jour
e tratamiento *m* psiquiátrico diurno;
tratamiento *m* psiquiátrico de día

i trattamento *m* psichiatrico diurno
n psychiatrische dagbehandeling
d psychiatrische Tagesbehandlung *f*

451 DAY RATE
see: COST PER DAY

452 DAY ROOM
f salle *f* de jour;
local *m* de jour;
salle *f* de séjour;
pièce *f* de séjour
e sala *f* diurna;
sala *f* de día
i sala *f* di soggiorno;
stanza *f* di soggiorno
n dagverblijf *n*
d Tagesraum *m*;
Aufenthaltsraum *m*

453 DAY TREATMENT
f traitement *m* de jour
e tratamiento *m* diurno;
tratamiento *m* de día
i trattamento *m* diurno
n dagbehandeling
d Tagesbehandlung *f*

454 DAY UNIT
f unité *f* de jour
e unidad *f* de cuidado diurno (atención diurna, asistencia diurna)
i unità *f* di cure diurne
n dageenheid
d Tagesstation *f*

455 DEAD BODY
see: CADAVER

456 DEATH RATE;
MORTALITY
f chiffre *m* des décès;
mortalité *f*
e cifra *f* de mortalidad;
mortalidad *f*
i numero *m* dei decessi;
mortalità *f*
n sterftecijfer *n*;
mortaliteit
d Sterblichkeitsziffer *f*;
Mortalität *f*

457 DEEP X-RAY THERAPY
f radiothérapie *f* pénétrante;
radiothérapie *f* profonde
e radioterapia *f* penetrante
i radioterapia *f* penetrante;
radioterapia *f* profonda
n röntgendieptetherapie
d Röntgentiefentherapie *f*

458 DELIVERY ROOM
f salle *f* d'accouchements
e sala *f* de maternidad;
sala *f* de partos
i sala *f* parto
n verloskamer
d Entbindungsraum *m*;
Entbindungszimmer *n*;
Kreissaal *m*

459 DEMAND FOR BEDS
see: BED NEED

460 DENTAL CARE
f soins *mpl* dentaires;
soins *mpl* des dents
e cuidado *m* dental;
cuidado *m* de los dientes
i cure *fpl* dentarie;
cure *fpl* dei denti
n tandverzorging
d Zahnpflege *f*

461 DENTAL CLINIC;
DENTISTRY CLINIC
f clinique *f* dentaire
e clínica *f* dental
i clinica *f* odontoiatrica
n tandheelkundige kliniek
d zahnärztliche Klinik *f*;
Zahnklinik *f*

462 DENTAL DEPARTMENT;
DENTISTRY DEPARTMENT
f service *m* (département *m*) dentaire
e servicio *m* (departamento *m*) dental
i divisione *f* odontoiatrica
n tandheelkundige afdeling
d zahnärztliche Abteilung *f*;
Zahnabteilung *f*

463 DENTAL HEALTH CARE
f soins *mpl* odontologiques
e asistencia *f* dental;
ayuda *f* dental
i cure *fpl* odontoiatriche
n tandheelkundige zorg;
tandheelkundige hulp
d zahnärztliche Fürsorge *f*

464 DENTAL HOSPITAL;
DENTISTRY HOSPITAL
f hôpital *m* dentaire
e hospital *m* dental
i ospedale *m* odontoiatrico
n tandheelkundig ziekenhuis *n*
d zahnärztliches Krankenhaus *n*

465 DENTAL HYGIENE
f hygiène *f* dentaire
e higiene *f* dental
i igiene *f* dentaria
n tandhygiëne
d Zahnhygiene *f*

466 DENTAL MECHANIC
f technicien *m* dentaire
e técnico *m* dentista
i odontotècnico *m*
n tandtechnicus
d Zahntechniker *m*

467 DENTAL SURGEON;
DENTIST;
SURGEON DENTIST
f dentiste *m*
e dentista *m*;
odontólogo *m*
i dentista *m*
n tandarts
d Zahnarzt *m*

468 DENTAL SURGERY
f chirurgie *f* dentaire
e cirugía *f* dental
i chirurgia *f* dentaria
n tandchirurgie
d Zahnchirurgie *f*

469 DENTAL TREATMENT
f traitement *m* dentaire
e tratamiento *m* dental
i trattamento *m* dentario
n tandheelkundige behandeling
d Zahnbehandlung *f*;
zahnärztliche Behandlung *f*

470 DENTAL UNIT;
DENTISTRY UNIT
f unité *f* dentaire
e unidad *f* dental
i unità *f* odontoiatrica
n tandheelkundige eenheid
d zahnärztliche Station *f*

471 DENTIST
see: DENTAL SURGEON

472 DENTISTRY
f odontologie *f*
e odontología *f*
i odontologia *f*
n tandheelkunde
d Zahnheilkunde *f*;
Zahnarzneikunst *f*

473 DENTISTRY CLINIC
see: DENTAL CLINIC

474 DENTISTRY DEPARTMENT
see: DENTAL DEPARTMENT

475 DENTISTRY HOSPITAL
see: DENTAL HOSPITAL

476 DENTISTRY UNIT
see: DENTAL UNIT

477 DERMATOLOGIST;
SKIN SPECIALIST
f dermatologiste *m*
e dermatólogo *m*;
especialista *m* para la piel
i dermatologo *m*
n dermatoloog;
huidarts;
huidspecialist
d Dermatologe *m*;
Hautarzt *m*;
Hautspezialist *m*

478 DERMATOLOGY
f dermatologie *f*
e dermatología *f*
i dermatologia *f*
n dermatologie
d Dermatologie *f*

479 DERMATOLOGY CLINIC;
SKIN DISEASES CLINIC
f clinique *f* dermatologique;
clinique *f* de dermatologie
e clínica *f* dermatológica;
clínica *f* de dermatología
i clinica *f* dermosifilopatica;
clinica *f* di dermosifilopatia
n dermatologische kliniek;
huidkliniek
d Hautklinik *f*

480 DERMATOLOGY DEPARTMENT;
SKIN DISEASES DEPARTMENT
f service *m* (département *m*) dermatologique;
service *m* (département *m*) de dermatologie
e servicio *m* (departamento *m*) dermatológico;
servicio *m* (departamento *m*) de dermatología
i divisione *f* dermosifilopatica;
divisione *f* di dermosifilopatia
n dermatologische afdeling;
huidafdeling
d Hautabteilung *f*

481 DERMATOLOGY HOSPITAL;
SKIN DISEASES HOSPITAL
f hôpital *m* dermatologique;
hôpital *m* de dermatologie
e hospital *m* dermatológico;
hospital *m* de dermatología
i ospedale *m* dermosifilopatico;
ospedale *m* di dermosifilopatia
n dermatologisch ziekenhuis *n*
d Hautkrankenhaus *n*

482 DERMATOLOGY UNIT;
SKIN DISEASES UNIT
f unité *f* dermatologique;
unité *f* de dermatologie
e unidad *f* dermatológica;
unidad *f* de dermatología
i unità *f* dermosifilopatica;
unità *f* di dermosifilopatia
n dermatologische eenheid
d Hautstation *f*

483 DIABETES
f diabète *m*
e diabetes *f*;
diabetis *f*
i diabete *m*
n diabetes
d Diabetes *m*

484 DIAGNOSIS
f diagnose *f*
e diagnosis *f*
i diagnosi *f*
n diagnose
d Diagnose *f*

485 DIAGNOSTIC CENTRE (CENTER)
f centre *m* de diagnostic
e centro *m* de diagnóstico
i centro *m* di diagnostica
n diagnosecentrum *n*
d Diagnosezentrum *n*;
Diagnostikzentrum *n*

486 DIAGNOSTIC CLINIC
f clinique *f* de diagnostic
e clínica *f* de diagnóstico
i clinica *f* di diagnostica
n diagnosekliniek
d Diagnoseklinik *f*

487 DIAGNOSTIC COMPUTER
f ordinateur *m* de diagnostic
e computadora *m* de diagnóstico

i compiuter *m* diagnostico
n diagnostische computer
d diagnostischer Komputer *m*

488 DIAGNOSTIC DEPARTMENT
f service *m* (département *m*) de diagnostic
e servicio *m* (departamento *m*) de diagnóstico
i servizio *m* di diagnostica
n diagnose-afdeling
d Diagnoseabteilung *f*

489 DIAGNOSTIC HOSPITAL
f hôpital *m* de diagnostic
e hospital *m* de diagnóstico
i ospedale *m* di diagnostica
n diagnoseziekenhuis *n*
d Diagnosekrankenhaus *n*

490 DIAGNOSTIC RADIOLOGICAL APPARATUS;
DIAGNOSTIC RADIOLOGY APPARATUS;
DIAGNOSTIC X-RAY APPARATUS
f appareils *mpl* radiologiques de diagnostic
e aparatos *mpl* radiológicos de diagnóstico
i apparecchi *mpl* radiologici di diagnosi
n diagnostische röntgenapparatuur
d diagnostische Röntgengeräte *npl*

491 DIAGNOSTIC RADIOLOGICAL DEPARTMENT;
DIAGNOSTIC RADIOLOGY DEPARTMENT;
DIAGNOSTIC X-RAY DEPARTMENT
f service *m* (département *m*) de radiologie diagnostique;
service *m* (département *m*) de radiodiagnostic
e servicio *m* (departamento *m*) de radiología de diagnóstico
i servizio *m* di radiodiagnostica
n röntgendiagnose-afdeling
d diagnostische Röntgenabteilung *f*;
röntgendiagnostische Abteilung *f*

492 DIAGNOSTIC RADIOLOGY
f radiologie *f* de diagnostic
e radiología *f* de diagnóstico
i radiologia *f* diagnostica
n diagnostische radiologie
d diagnostische Radiologie *f*

493 DIAGNOSTIC RADIOLOGY APPARATUS
see: DIAGNOSTIC RADIOLOGICAL APPARATUS

494 DIAGNOSTIC RADIOLOGY DEPARTMENT
see: DIAGNOSTIC RADIOLOGICAL DEPARTMENT

495 DIAGNOSTIC UNIT
f unité *f* de diagnostic
e unidad *f* de diagnóstico
i unità *f* di diagnostica
n diagnose-eenheid
d Diagnosestation *f*

496 DIAGNOSTIC X-RAY APPARATUS
see: DIAGNOSTIC RADIOLOGICAL APPARATUS

497 DIAGNOSTIC X-RAY DEPARTMENT
see: DIAGNOSTIC RADIOLOGICAL DEPARTMENT

498 DIALYSIS APPARATUS
f appareils *mpl* de dialyse
e aparatos *mpl* de diálisis
i apparecchi *mpl* per dialisi
n dialyse-apparatuur
d Dialysegeräte *npl*

499 DIALYSIS UNIT
f unité *f* de dialyse
e unidad *f* de diálisis
i unità *f* di dialisi
n dialyse-eenheid
d Dialysestation *f*

500 DIET
f régime *m*
e dieta *f*
i regime *m*
n dieet *n*
d Diät *n*

501 DIETARY DEPARTMENT;
DIETETIC DEPARTMENT
f service *m* (département *m*) diététique
e servicio *m* (departamento *m*) dietético;
servicio *m* (departamento *m*) de dietética
i servizio *m* di dietetica
n dieetafdeling
d Diätabteilung *f*

502 DIETARY UNIT;
DIETETIC UNIT
f unité *f* diététique
e unidad *f* dietética;
unidad *f* de dietética
i unità *f* di dietetica
n dieeteenheid
d Diätstation *f*

503 DIETETIC DEPARTMENT
see: DIETARY DEPARTMENT

504 DIETETICS
f diététique *f*
e dietética *f*
i dietetica *f*
n diëtetiek
d Diätetik *f*

505 DIETETIC UNIT
see: DIETARY UNIT

506 DIETICIAN;
DIETIST;
DIETITIAN
f diétiste *m*
e dietista *m*
i dietista *m*
n diëtist
d Diätist *m*

507 DIETIST
see: DIETICIAN

508 DIETITIAN
see: DIETICIAN

509 DIETKITCHEN
f cuisine *f* diététique
e cocina *f* dietética
i cucina *f* dietetica
n dieetkeuken
d Diätküche *f*

510 DIETTHERAPY
f thérapie *f* diététique
e terapia *f* dietética
i terapia *f* dietetica
n dieettherapie
d Diättherapie *f*

511 DIPLOMA NURSE;
GRADUATE NURSE;
REGISTERED NURSE
f infirmière *f* diplômée
e enfermera *f* diplomada
i infermiera *f* diplomata
n gediplomeerde verpleegkundige;
gediplomeerde verplegende;
gediplomeerde verpleegster
d Diplom-Krankenschwester *f*;
diplomierte Krankenschwester *f*

512 DIRECTOR OF NURSING
see: CHIEF NURSING OFFICER

513 DIRECTOR OF NURSING SERVICE
see: CHIEF NURSING OFFICER

514 DISABLEMENT INSURANCE;
INVALIDITY INSURANCE
f assurance-invalidité *f*;
assurance *f* contre l'invalidité
e seguro *m* de invalidez;
seguro *m* contra invalidez
i assicurazione *f* invalidità;
assicurazione *f* contro l'invalidità
n invaliditeitsverzekering
d Invaliditätsversicherung *f*

515 DISCHARGE;
INPATIENT DISCHARGE
f décharge *f*;
démission *f*;
sortie *f*;
licenciement *m*
e egreso *m*;
salida *f*;
alta *f*;
despido *m*
i dimissione *f*;
uscita *f*
n ontslag *n*
d Entlassung *f*

516 DISCHARGE DAY
f jour *m* de décharge
e día *m* de egreso
i giorno *m* dell'uscita
n ontslagdag
d Entlassungstag *m*

517 DISCHARGE INTERVIEW;
EXIT INTERVIEW
f interview *f* de sortie
e entrevista *f* de egreso
i intervista *f* di dimissione
n exit interview *n*
d Entlassungsinterview *n*

518 DISCHARGE PROCEDURE
f procédure *f* de décharge
e procedimiento *m* de egreso
i procedura *f* di dimissione
n ontslagprocedure
d Entlassungsverfahren *n*

519 DISCHARGE SERVICE
f service *m* de décharge
e servicio *m* de egreso
i servizio *m* di dimissione
n ontslagdienst
d Entlassungsdienst *m*

520 DISCHARGE STATISTICS
f statistique *f* de décharge
e estadística *f* de egreso
i statistica *f* delle dimissioni
n ontslagstatistiek
d Entlassungsstatistik *f*

521 DISEASE;
ILLNESS;
SICKNESS
f maladie *f*
e enfermedad *f*
i malattia *f*
n ziekte
d Krankheit *f*

522 DISEASE CLASSIFICATION;
ILLNESS CLASSIFICATION
f classification *f* des maladies
e clasificación *f* de enfermedades
i classificazione *f* delle malattie
n ziekteclassificatie
d Krankheitsklassifikation *f*

523 DISEASE PREVENTION;
ILLNESS PREVENTION
f prévention *f* des maladies
e prevención *f* de enfermedades
i prevenzione *f* delle malattie
n ziektepreventie;
voorkoming van ziekte
d Krankheitsvorbeugung *f*;
Krankheitsverhütung *f*

524 DISEASE TRANSMISSION;
ILLNESS TRANSMISSION
f transmission *f* des maladies
e transmisión *f* de enfermedades
i trasmissione *f* delle malattie
n ziekte-overbrenging
d Krankheitsübertragung *f*

525 DISINFECTANT STORE
f dépôt *m* de produits désinfectants
e depósito *m* para desinfectantes
i deposito *m* dei disinfettanti
n berging voor desinfecterende middelen
d Lager *n* für Desinfektionsmittel

526 DISINFECTING APPARATUS
f appareils *mpl* de désinfection
e aparatos *mpl* de desinfección
i apparecchi *mpl* per disinfezione
n desinfectie-apparatuur
d Desinfektionsgeräte *npl*

527 DISINFECTION
f désinfection *f*
e desinfección *f*
i disinfezione *f*
n desinfectie
d Desinfektion *f*

528 DISTRICT GENERAL HOSPITAL
f hôpital *m* général de district;
hôpital *m* général de zone
e hospital *m* general de distrito
i ospedale *m* generale di zona
n algemeen streekziekenhuis *n*
d allgemeines Bezirkskrankenhaus *n*;
allgemeines Bezirksspital *n*;
allgemeines Kreiskrankenhaus *n*;
allgemeines Kreisspital *n*

529 DISTRICT NURSE;
VISITING NURSE
f infirmière *f* visiteuse;
infirmière *f* visitante
e enfermera *f* del barrio
i assistente *f* visitatrice sanitaria
n wijkverpleegster;
wijkverpleegkundige;
wijkverplegende
d Gemeindeschwester *f*

530 DISTRICT NURSING
f soins *mpl* infirmiers de quartier
e enfermería *f* del barrio
i assistenza *f* infermieristica di quartiere
n wijkverpleging
d Gemeindepflege *f*

531 DOCTOR;
MEDICAL PRACTITIONER;
PHYSICIAN
f médecin *m*
e médico *m*;
doctor *m*
i medico *m*
n arts
d Arzt *m*

532 DOCTORS' COUNCIL
f conseil *m* des médecins
e consejo *m* de los médicos
i consiglio *m* dei medici
n medische staf
d Ärztebeirat *m*

533 DOCTOR'S FEE;
MEDICAL FEE
f honoraires *mpl* de médecin;
honoraires *mpl* médicaux
e honorarios *mpl* del médico;
honorarios *mpl* médicos
i onorario *m* del medico;
onorario *m* medico
n artsenhonorarium *n*
d Arzthonorar *n*;
ärztliches Honorar *n*

534 DOCTOR'S PRACTICE
f cabinet *m* de médecin
e práctica *f* médica
i gabinetto *m* medico
n artsenpraktijk
d Arztpraxis *f*

535 DOCTORS' QUARTER;
MEDICAL STAFF ROOM
f bureau *m* pour médecins
e cuarto *m* para los médicos
i ufficio *m* per medici
n artsenkamer
d Arztzimmer *n*

536 DOMICILIARY CARE;
HOME CARE;
HOME HEALTH CARE
f soins *mpl* à domicile;
soins *mpl* sanitaires à domicile
e cuidado *m* domiciliario;
cuidado *m* a domicilio;
atención *f* domiciliaria;
atención *f* a domicilio
i cure *fpl* domiciliari;
assistenza *f* domiciliare
n thuisverzorging;
thuiszorg
d Heimversorgung *f*

537 DOMICILIARY NURSING;
HOME NURSING
f soins *mpl* infirmiers à domicile
e enfermería *f* domiciliaria;
enfermería *f* a domicilio
i assistenza *f* infermieristica a domicilio
n thuisverpleging
d Haus(kranken)pflege *f*;
Heimpflege *f*;
häusliche Pflege *f*

538 DRESSING ROOM
f salle *f* de pansement
e sala *f* de vendaje
i sala *f* di medicazione
n verbandkamer
d Verbandszimmer *n*

539 DRUG;
MEDICINE;
REMEDY
f médicament *m*;
remède *m*
e medicina *f*;
remedio *m*;
medicamento *m*
i medicamento *m*
n geneesmiddel *n*;
medicijn;
medicament *n*
d Arzneimittel *n*;
Arznei *f*;
Medikament *n*;
Heilmittel *n*

540 DRUG ADDICT
f toxicomane *m*
e toxicómano *m*
i tossicomane *m*
n verslaafde aan verdovende middelen
d Rauschgiftsüchtiger *m*

541 DRUG ADDICTION
f toxicomanie *f*
e toxicomanía *f*
i tossicomania *f*
n verslaafdheid aan verdovende middelen
d Rauschgiftsucht *f*

542 DRUGS ADMINISTRATION
f administration *f* des médicaments
e administración *f* de medicinas
i somministrazione *f* di medicamenti
n geneesmiddelentoediening
d Arzneimittelverabreichung *f*

543 DRUGS CONSUMPTION
f consommation *f* pharmaceutique;
consommation *f* des médicaments
e consumo *m* farmacéutico;
consumo *m* de medicinas
i consumo *m* farmaceutico;
consumo *m* di medicinali
n geneesmiddelenverbruik *n*
d Arzneimittelverbrauch *m*

544 DRUGS CONTROL
f contrôle *m* des médicaments
e comprobación *f* de medicinas;
control *m* de medicinas
i controllo *m* dei medicinali
n geneesmiddelencontrole
d Arzneimittelkontrolle *f*

545 DRUGS DISTRIBUTION
f distribution *f* des médicaments
e distribución *f* de medicinas
i distribuzione *f* dei medicinali
n geneesmiddelendistributie
d Arzneimittelverteilung *f*

546 DRUGS INFORMATION
f information *f* pharmaceutique
e información *f* farmacéutica
i informazione *f* farmaceutica
n geneesmiddeleninformatie
d Arzneimittelinformation *f*

547 DRUGS PRESCRIBING
f prescription *f* des médicaments
e prescripción *f* de medicinas
i prescrizione *f* dei medicinali
n voorschrijven *n* van geneesmiddelen
d Arzneimittelverordnung *f*

548 DRUGS STORE
f magasin *m* pour médicaments
e almacén *m* para medicinas
i deposito *m* dei medicinali
n geneesmiddelenmagazijn *n*
d Arzneimittellager *n*

549 DRUGS SUPPLY
f approvisionnement *m* en médicaments;
ravitaillement *m* en médicaments
e suministro *m* de medicinas
i scorta *f* dei medicinali
n geneesmiddelenvoorziening
d Arzneimittelversorgung *f*

550 DURATION OF HOSPITALIZATION;
DURATION OF HOSPITAL STAY;
DURATION OF INPATIENT HOSPITALIZATION;
DURATION OF STAY;
HOSPITALIZATION LENGTH;
HOSPITALIZATION TIME;
LENGTH OF HOSPITALIZATION;
LENGTH OF STAY;
STAY LENGTH
f durée *f* de l'hospitalisation;
durée *f* de séjour
e duración *f* de la hospitalización;
duración *f* de la estancia;
duración *f* de la estadía
i durata *f* del soggiorno
n verpleegduur;
ligduur;
verblijfsduur;
opnameduur
d Verweildauer *f*;
Pflegedauer *f*;
Aufenthaltsdauer *f*;
Liegedauer *f*;
Liegezeit *f*

551 DURATION OF HOSPITAL STAY
see: DURATION OF HOSPITALIZATION

552 DURATION OF INPATIENT HOSPITALIZATION
see: DURATION OF HOSPITALIZATION

553 DURATION OF STAY
see: DURATION OF HOSPITALIZATION

554 DYING PATIENT;
TERMINAL CARE PATIENT;
TERMINAL PATIENT
f malade *m* (patient *m*) mourant;
malade *m* (patient *m*) moribond
e paciente *m* (enfermo *m*) moribundo
i malato *m* moribondo
n stervende patiënt;
terminale patiënt
d sterbender Patient *m* (Kranker *m*)

E

555 EAR BANK
f banque *f* d'oreilles
e banco *m* de orejas
i banca *f* delle orecchie
n oorbank
d Ohrenbank *f*

556 EAR, NOSE AND THROAT CLINIC;
ENT CLINIC
f clinique *f* d'oto-rhino-laryngologie;
clinique *f* d'ORL
e clínica *f* de oído nariz y garganta
i clinica *f* di otorinolaringoiatria;
clinica *f* d'ORL
n keel- neus- en oorheelkundige kliniek;
KNO-kliniek
d Hals- Nasen- und Ohrenklinik *f*;
HNO-Klinik *f*

557 EAR, NOSE AND THROAT DEPARTMENT;
ENT DEPARTMENT
f service *m* (département *m*) d'oto-rhino-laryngologie;
service *m* (département *m*) d'ORL
e servicio *m* (departamento *m*) de oído nariz y garganta
i divisione *f* di otorinolaringoiatria;
divisione *f* d'ORL
n keel- neus- en oorheelkundige afdeling;
KNO-afdeling
d Hals- Nasen- und Ohrenabteilung *f*;
HNO-Abteilung *f*

558 EAR, NOSE AND THROAT DISEASE
f maladie *f* de gorge de nez et d'oreille;
maladie *f* ORL
e enfermedad *f* de oído nariz y garganta
i malattia *f* otorinolaringoiatrica;
malattia *f* ORL
n keel- neus- en oorziekte
d Hals- Nasen- und Ohrenkrankheit *f*

559 EAR, NOSE AND THROAT HOSPITAL;
ENT HOSPITAL
f hôpital *m* d'oto-rhino-laryngologie;
hôpital *m* d'ORL
e hospital *m* de oído nariz y garganta
i ospedale *m* di otorinolaringoiatria;
ospedale *m* ORL
n keel- neus- en oorheelkundig ziekenhuis *n*;
KNO-ziekenhuis *n*
d Hals- Nasen- und Ohrenkrankenhaus *n*;
HNO-Krankenhaus *n*

560 EAR, NOSE AND THROAT INSTRUMENTS;
ENT INSTRUMENTS
f instruments *mpl* de gorge de nez et d'oreille
e instrumentos *mpl* para el oído la nariz y la garganta
i strumenti *mpl* per gola naso e orecchi
n keel- neus- en oorinstrumenten
d Hals- Nasen- und Ohreninstrumente *npl*

561 EAR, NOSE AND THROAT PHYSICIAN;
EAR, NOSE AND THROAT SPECIALIST;
ENT PHYSICIAN;
ENT SPECIALIST
f oto-rhino-laryngologiste *m*
e otorrinolaringólogo *m*;
especialista *m* para el oído la nariz y la garganta
i otorinolaringoiatra *m*
n keel- neus- en oorarts;
KNO-arts
d Hals- Nasen- und Ohrenarzt *m*;
HNO-Arzt *m*

562 EAR, NOSE AND THROAT SPECIALIST
see: EAR, NOSE AND THROAT PHYSICIAN

563 EAR, NOSE AND THROAT UNIT;
ENT UNIT
f unité *f* d'oto-rhino-laryngologie;
unité *f* d'ORL
e unidad *f* de oído nariz y garganta
i unità *f* di otorinolaringoiatria;
unità *f* d'ORL
n keel- neus- en oorheelkundige eenheid;
KNO-eenheid
d Hals- Nasen- und Ohrenstation *f*;
HNO-Station *f*

564 ECG
see: ELECTROCARDIOGRAPHY

565 ECOLOGY
f écologie *f*
e ecología *f*
i ecologia *f*
n ecologie
d Ekologie *f*

566 EEG
see: ELECTROENCEPHALOGRAPHY

567 ELECTROCARDIOGRAPHY;
ECG
f électrocardiographie *f*;
ECG *f*
e electrocardiografía *f*;
ECG *f*
i elettrocardiografia *f*;
ECG *f*
n electrocardiografie;
ECG
d Elektrokardiographie *f*;
EKG *f*

568 ELECTROCARDIOGRAPHY ROOM
f salle *f* d'électrocardiographie
e sala *f* de electrocardiografía
i sala *f* per elettrocardiografia
n electrocardiografieruimte
d Raum *m* für Elektrokardiographie

569 ELECTROCARDIOLOGY
f électrocardiologie *f*
e electrocardiología *f*
i elettrocardiologia *f*
n electrocardiologie
d Elektrokardiologie *f*

570 ELECTROENCEPHALOGRAPHY;
EEG
f électroencéphalographie *f*;
EEG *f*

e electroencefalografía *f*;
EEG *f*
i elettroencefalografia *f*;
EEG *f*
n electro-encefalografie;
EEG
d Elektroenzephalographie *f*;
EEG *f*

571 ELECTROENCEPHALOGRAPHY ROOM
f salle *f* d'électroencéphalographie
e sala *f* de electroencefalografía
i sala *f* per elettroencefalografia
n electro-encefalografieruimte
d Raum *m* für Elektroenzephalographie

572 ELECTRO-MEDICAL APPARATUS
f appareils *mpl* électro-médicaux
e aparatos *mpl* electro-médicos
i apparecchi *mpl* elettrici sanitari
n electromedische apparatuur
d elektromedizinische Geräte *npl*

573 ELECTROTHERAPY
f électrothérapie *f*
e electroterapia *f*
i elettroterapia *f*
n electrotherapie
d Elektrotherapie *f*

574 ELECTROTHERAPY ROOM
f salle *f* d'électrothérapie
e sala *f* de electroterapia
i sala *f* d'elettroterapia
n electrotherapieruimte
d Raum *m* für Elektrotherapie

575 EMERGENCY ADMISSION
f admission *f* d'urgence
e admisión *f* de urgencia;
admisión *f* de emergencia
i ricovero *m* d'urgenza
n spoedopneming
d Notaufnahme *f*;
Aufnahme *f* dringlicher Fälle

576 EMERGENCY AID
f aide *f* d'urgence;
secours *m* d'urgence
e ayuda *f* inmediata
i aiuto *m* d'urgenza
n onmiddellijke hulpverlening;
spoedeisende hulp
d Soforthilfe *f*

577 EMERGENCY AMBULANCE
f ambulance *f* d'urgence
e ambulancia *f* de urgencia;
ambulancia *f* de emergencia
i ambulanza *f* d'urgenza
n spoedambulance
d Notambulanz *f*

578 EMERGENCY BED
f lit *m* d'urgence
e cama *f* para casos urgentes
i letto *m* d'urgenza
n bed *n* voor spoedgevallen
d Notfallbett *n*;
Bett *n* für dringliche Fälle

579 EMERGENCY CARE
f soins *mpl* d'urgence
e cuidado *m* (atención *f*) de urgencia;
cuidado *m* (atención *f*) de emergencia
i cure *fpl* d'urgenza
n spoedgevallenzorg
d Notfallversorgung *f*;
Nothilfe *f*

580 EMERGENCY CENTRE (CENTER)
f centre *m* d'urgence
e centro *m* de urgencia;
centro *m* de emergencia
i centro *m* di pronto soccorso
n spoedgevallencentrum *n*
d Notbehandlungszentrum *n*;
Zentrum *n* für dringliche Fälle

581 EMERGENCY CLINIC
f clinique *f* d'urgence
e clínica *f* de urgencia;
clínica *f* de emergencia
i clinica *f* di pronto soccorso
n kliniek voor spoedgevallen
d Notfallklinik *f*;
Klinik *f* für dringliche Fälle

582 EMERGENCY DEPARTMENT
f service *m* (département *m*) d'urgence
e servicio *m* (departamento *m*) de urgencia;
servicio *m* (departamento *m*) de emergencia
i servizio *m* di urgenza
n spoedgevallenafdeling;
spoedhulpafdeling;
afdeling voor spoedeisende hulp
d Notfallabteilung *f*;
Nothilfeabteilung *f*;
Abteilung *f* für dringliche Fälle

583 EMERGENCY HEALTH TRANSPORT
f transport *m* sanitaire d'urgence
e transporte *m* sanitario de urgencia;
transporte *m* sanitario de emergencia
i trasporto *m* sanitario d'urgenza
n spoedgevallentransport *n*
d Transport *m* von Notfallpatienten

584 EMERGENCY HOSPITAL
f hôpital *m* d'urgence
e hospital *m* de urgencia;
hospital *m* de emergencia
i ospedale *m* di pronto soccorso
n ziekenhuis *n* voor spoedgevallen
d Notfallkrankenhaus *n*

585 EMERGENCY MEDICAL CARE
f soins *mpl* médicaux d'urgence
e cuidado *m* médico de urgencia;
atención *f* médica de urgencia;
cuidado *m* médico de emergencia;
atención *f* médica de emergencia
i cure *fpl* mediche urgenti
n spoedeisende medische zorg
d ärztliche Versorgung *f* dringlicher Fälle

586 EMERGENCY MEDICINE
f médecine *f* d'urgence
e medicina *f* de urgencia;
medicina *f* de emergencia
i medicina *f* d'urgenza
n spoedgevallengeneeskunde;
noodgevallengeneeskunde
d Notfallmedizin *f*

587 EMERGENCY OBSTETRIC CARE
f soins *mpl* obstétricaux d'urgence
e cuidado *m* obstétrico de urgencia;
atención *f* obstétrica de urgencia;
cuidado *m* obstétrico de emergencia;
atención *f* obstétrica de emergencia
i cure *fpl* ostetriche d'urgenza
n onmiddellijke verloskundige zorg
d dringliche Geburtshilfe *f*

588 EMERGENCY SURGERY
f chirurgie *f* d'urgence
e cirugía *f* de urgencia;
cirugía *f* de emergencia
i chirurgia *f* d'urgenza
n chirurgie voor spoedgevallen
d Notfallchirurgie *f*

589 EMERGENCY TREATMENT
f traitement *m* d'urgence
e tratamiento *m* de urgencia;
tratamiento *m* de emergencia
i trattamento *m* d'urgenza
n spoedgevallenbehandeling
d Notfallbehandlung *f*

590 EMERGENCY UNIT
f unité *f* d'urgence
e unidad *f* de urgencia;
unidad *f* de emergencia
i unità *f* di pronto soccorso
n spoedgevalleneenheid
d Notfallstation *f*

591 ENDOCRINOLOGIC CLINIC
f clinique *f* d'endocrinologie
e clínica *f* endocrinológica;
clínica *f* de endocrinología
i clinica *f* endocrinologica
n endocrinologische kliniek
d Klinik *f* für Endokrinologie

592 ENDOCRINOLOGIST
f endocrinologiste *m*
e endocrinólogo *m*
i endocrinologo *m*
n endocrinoloog
d Endokrinologe *m*

593 ENDOCRINOLOGY
f endocrinologie *f*
e endocrinología *f*
i endocrinologia *f*
n endocrinologie
d Endokrinologie *f*

594 ENDOSCOPE
f endoscope *m*
e endoscopio *m*
i endoscopio *m*
n endoscoop
d Endoskop *n*

595 ENDOSCOPY
f endoscopie *f*
e endoscopia *f*
i endoscopia *f*
n endoscopie
d Endoskopie *f*

596 ENDOSCOPY DEPARTMENT
f service *m* (département *m*) d'endoscopie
e servicio *m* (departamento *m*) de endoscopia
i servizio *m* d'endoscopia
n endoscopie-afdeling
d endoskopische Abteilung *f*

597 ENT CLINIC
see: EAR, NOSE AND THROAT CLINIC

598 ENT DEPARTMENT
see: EAR, NOSE AND THROAT DEPARTMENT

599 ENT HOSPITAL
see: EAR, NOSE AND THROAT HOSPITAL

600 ENT INSTRUMENTS
see: EAR, NOSE AND THROAT INSTRUMENTS

601 ENT PHYSICIAN
see: EAR, NOSE AND THROAT PHYSICIAN

602 FNT SPECIALIST
see: EAR, NOSE AND THROAT PHYSICIAN

603 ENT UNIT
see: EAR, NOSE AND THROAT UNIT

604 ENVIRONMENTAL HEALTH;
ENVIRONMENTAL HYGIENE
f hygiène *f* du milieu;
hygiène *f* de l'environnement
e higiene *f* ambiental
i igiene *f* dell' ambiente
n milieuhygiëne
d Umwelthygiene *f*

605 ENVIRONMENTAL HYGIENE
see: ENVIRONMENTAL HEALTH

606 ENVIRONMENTAL MEDICINE
f médecine *f* du milieu;
médecine *f* de l'environnement
e medicina *f* ambiental
i medicina *f* dell' ambiente
n milieugeneeskunde
d Umweltmedizin *f*

607 ENVIRONMENTAL POLLUTION
f pollution *f* du milieu;
pollution *f* de l'environnement
e ensuciamiento *m* ambiental
i inquinamento *m* dell' ambiente
n milieuvervuiling
d Umweltverschmutzung *f*

608 ENVIRONMENTAL PROTECTION
f protection *f* du milieu;
protection *f* de l'environnement
e protección *f* ambiental
i protezione *f* dell' ambiente
n milieubescherming
d Umweltschutz *m*

609 EPIDEMICS CONTROL
f lutte *f* contre les épidémies
e lucha *f* antiepidémica;
lucha *f* contra epidemias
i lotta *f* contro le epidemie
n bestrijding van epidemieën
d Seuchenbekämpfung *f*

610 EPILEPSY CENTRE (CENTER)
f centre *m* pour épileptiques

e centro *m* para epilépticos
i centro *m* per epilettici
n epilepsiecentrum *n*
d Epilepsiezentrum *n*

611 EPILEPSY CLINIC
f clinique *f* pour épileptiques
e clínica *f* para epilépticos
i clinica *f* per epilettici
n epilepsiekliniek
d Epilepsieklinik *f*

612 EPILEPTIC CARE
f soins *mpl* aux épileptiques
e cuidado *m* (atención *f*) de los epilépticos;
asistencia *f* a los epilépticos
i trattamento *m* degli epilettici
n zorg voor epileptici
d Versorgung *f* von Epileptikern

613 ERGOTHERAP(EUT)IST;
WORK THERAP(EUT)IST
f ergothérapeute *m*
e terapeuta *m* por el trabajo
i ergoterapeuta *m*
n arbeidstherapeut
d Arbeitstherapeut *m*

614 ERGOTHERAPY;
WORK THERAPY
f ergothérapie *f*;
ergothérapeutique *f*;
thérapie *f* par le travail;
thérapeutique *f* par le travail
e ergoterapia *f*;
laborterapia *f*;
terapia *f* de (por) trabajo;
terapéutica *f* de (por) trabajo
i ergoterapia *f*
n ergotherapie;
arbeidstherapie
d Ergotherapie *f*;
Arbeitstherapie *f*

615 ERGOTHERAPY DEPARTMENT;
WORK THERAPY DEPARTMENT
f service *m* (département *m*) d'ergothérapie
e servicio *m* (departamento *m*) de ergoterapia
i servizio *m* di ergoterapia
n arbeidstherapeutische afdeling
d Abteilung *f* für Arbeitstherapie

616 EUTHANASIA
f euthanasie *f*
e eutanasia *f*
i eutanasia *f*
n euthanasie
d Euthanasie *f*

617 EXAMINATION ROOM
f salle *f* d'examens;
local *m* d'examens
e sala *f* de examen;
cuarto *m* de examen
i sala *f* di esame
n onderzoekkamer
d Untersuchungszimmer *n*;
Untersuchungsraum *m*

618 EXAMINATION TABLE
f table *f* d'examen
e mesa *f* de examen
i tavola *f* d'esame
n onderzoektafel
d Untersuchungstisch *m*

619 EXCRETA LABORATORY
see: COPROLOGICAL LABORATORY

620 EXERCISE POOL;
TREATMENT POOL
f piscine *f* de rééducation
e piscina *f* de revalidación
i piscina *f* di rieducazione
n oefenbad *n*
d Behandlungsbad *n*

621 EXIT INTERVIEW
see: DISCHARGE INTERVIEW

622 EXTENDED CARE;
POST-HOSPITAL CARE
f soins *mpl* post-hospitaliers
e cuidado *m* post-hospitalario;
atención *f* post-hospitalaria
i cure *fpl* post-ospedaliere
n ziekenhuisnazorg
d Pflege *f* nach einem Krankenhausaufenthalt;
Nachbetreuung *f*

623 EXTENDED CARE FACILITIES
f services *mpl* de soins post-hospitaliers
e servicios *mpl* de cuidado post-hospitalario (atención post-hospitalaria)
i servizi *mpl* de cure post-ospedaliere
n voorzieningen voor ziekenhuisnazorg
d Nachbetreuungsdienste *mpl*

624 EXTENDED CARE INSTITUTION
f établissement *m* de soins post-hospitaliers
e institución *f* de cuidado post-hospitalario (atención post-hospitalaria)
i istituto *m* di cure post-ospedaliere
n inrichting voor ziekenhuisnazorg
d Nachbetreuungsanstalt *f*

625 EXTRAMURAL CARE;
NON-INSTITUTIONAL CARE
f soins *mpl* extra-hospitaliers;
soins *mpl* extra-muros
e cuidado *m* extra-hospitalario;
atención *f* (asistencia *f*) extra-hospitalaria;
cuidado *m* (atención *f*, asistencia *f*) para-institucional
i cure *fpl* extra-ospedaliere;
assistenza *f* extra-ospedaliera
n extramurale zorg
d extramurale Fürsorge *f*;
extramurale Pflege *f*;
extramurale Betreuung *f*;
extramurale Versorgung *f*

626 EXTRAMURAL FACILITIES;
NON-INSTITUTIONAL FACILITIES
f services *mpl* extra-hospitaliers
e servicios *mpl* extra-hospitalarios;
servicios *mpl* para-institucionales
i servizi *mpl* extra-ospedalieri
n extramurale voorzieningen
d Aussendienste *mpl*;
extramurale Dienste *mpl*

627 EXTRAMURAL HEALTH CARE;
NON-INSTITUTIONAL HEALTH CARE
f soins *mpl* sanitaires extra-hospitaliers;

soins *mpl* sanitaires extra-muros;
soins *mpl* sanitaires sans placement
e cuidado *m* sanitario extra-hospitalario;
atención *f* (asistencia *f*) sanitaria extra-hospitalaria;
cuidado *m* sanitario para-institucional;
atención *f* (asistencia *f*) sanitaria para-institucional
i cure *fpl* sanitarie extra-ospedaliere;
assistenza *f* sanitaria extra-ospedaliera
n extramurale gezondheidszorg
d offene Gesundheitsfürsorge *f*;
extramurale Gesundheitsfürsorge *f*

628 EXTRAMURAL HEALTH FACILITIES;
NON-INSTITUTIONAL HEALTH FACILITIES
f services *mpl* sanitaires extra-hospitaliers;
services *mpl* sanitaires extra-muros;
services *mpl* sanitaires sans placement
e servicios *mpl* sanitarios extra-hospitalarios;
servicios *mpl* sanitarios para-institucionales
i servizi *mpl* sanitari extra-ospedalieri
n extramurale gezondheidsvoorzieningen
d offene Gesundheitsfürsorgedienste *mpl*;
extramurale Gesundheitsfürsorgedienste *mpl*

629 EYE BANK
f banque *f* d'yeux
e banco *m* de ojos
i banca *f* degli occhi
n oogbank
d Augenbank *f*

630 EYE CLINIC;
OPHTHALMIC CLINIC;
OPHTHALMOLOGY CLINIC
f clinique *f* ophtalmologique;
clinique *f* d'ophtalmologie
e clínica *f* oftalmológica
i clinica *f* oculistica
n oogkliniek
d Augenklinik *f*

631 EYE DEPARTMENT;
OPHTHALMIC DEPARTMENT;
OPHTHALMOLOGY DEPARTMENT
f service *m* (département *m*) ophtalmologique;
service *m* (département *m*) d'ophtalmologie
e servicio *m* (departamento *m*) oftalmológico
i divisione *f* oculistica
n oogafdeling
d Augenabteilung *f*

632 EYE HOSPITAL;
OPHTHALMIC HOSPITAL;
OPHTHALMOLOGY HOSPITAL
f hôpital *m* ophtalmologique;
hôpital *m* d'ophtalmologie
e hospital *m* oftalmológico
i ospedale *m* oculistico
n oogziekenhuis *n*
d Augenkrankenhaus *n*

633 EYE SPECIALIST;
OCULIST;
OPHTHALMOLOGIST
f oculiste *m*;
ophtalmologiste *m*;
ophtalmologue *m*
e oculista *m*;
oftalmólogo *m*
i oculista *m*
n oogarts;
oogheelkundige
d Augenarzt *m*

634 EYE SURGERY;
OPHTHALMIC SURGERY
f chirurgie *f* ophtalmique
e cirugía *f* oftálmica;
cirugía *f* del ojo
i chirurgia *f* oftalmica
n oogchirurgie
d Augenchirurgie *f*

635 EYE UNIT;
OPHTHALMIC UNIT;
OPHTHALMOLOGY UNIT
f unité *f* ophtalmologique;
unité *f* d'ophtalmologie
e unidad *f* oftalmológica
i unità *f* oculistica
n oogeenheid
d Augenstation *f*

F

636 FACTORY PHYSICIAN;
INDUSTRIAL PHYSICIAN;
OCCUPATIONAL PHYSICIAN;
PLANT PHYSICIAN
f médecin *m* d'entreprise;
médecin *m* d'usine;
médecin *m* du travail
e médico *m* de empresa;
médico *m* laboral
i medico *m* interno di un'impresa
n bedrijfsarts;
arbeidsarts
d Gewerbearzt *m*;
Betriebsarzt *m*;
Werksarzt *m*

637 FAMILY CARE
f soins *mpl* en famille
e cuidado *m* (atención *f*) familiar
i cure *fpl* in famiglia
n gezinszorg;
gezinsverpleging
d Familien(kranken)pflege *f*

638 FAMILY DOCTOR;
FAMILY PHYSICIAN;
GENERALIST;
GENERAL PRACTITIONER
f médecin *m* de famille;
médecin *m* généraliste;
généraliste *m*;
médecin *m* practicien;
omnipracticien *m*;
médecin *m* de médecine générale
e médico *m* de cabecera;
médico *m* de familia;
médico *m* de casa
i medico *m* di famiglia;
medico *m* generico
n huisarts;
familie-arts
d Hausarzt *m*;
praktischer Arzt *m*;
Allgemeinpraktiker *m*;
Familiendoktor *m*

639 FAMILY MEDICINE
f médecine *f* familiale
e medicina *f* familiar
i medicina *f* familiare
n gezinsgeneeskunde
d Familienmedizin *f*

640 FAMILY PHYSICIAN
see: FAMILY DOCTOR

641 FAMILY PLANNING
f planning *m* familial
e planificación *f* familiar;
planificación *f* de familia
i pianificazione *f* familiare
n gezinsplanning
d Familienplanung *f*

642 FAMILY PSYCHIATRY
f psychiatrie *f* familiale
e psiquiatría *f* familiar
i psichiatria *f* familiare
n gezinspsychiatrie
d Familienpsychiatrie *f*

643 FEVER THERAPY
f thérapie *f* de fièvre
e terapia *f* de fiebre
i terapia *f* mediante la febbre
n koortstherapie
d Fiebertherapie *f*

644 FIELD-HOSPITAL
f ambulance *f*
e hospital *m* de sangre;
enfermería *f* de campaña;
ambulancia *f*
i ambulanza *f*
n veldhospitaal; *n*
ambulance
d Feldlazarett *n*;
Feldhospital *n*

645 FIRST AID
f prompts secours *mpl*;
premiers soins *mpl*
e primeros auxilios *mpl*;
primera cura *f*
i primi soccorsi *mpl*;
prime cure *fpl*
n eerste hulp (bij ongelukken);
E.H.B.O.
d erste Hilfe *f*

646 FIRST AID SERVICES
f services *mpl* de prompts secours
e servicios *mpl* de primeros auxilios
i servizi *mpl* di pronto soccorso
n E.H.B.O.-diensten
d Dienste *mpl* für erste Hilfe

647 FLOOR KITCHEN;
WARD KITCHEN
f cuisine *f* relais;
cuisine *f* d'étage
e cocina *f* departamental
i cucina *f* di reparto
n afdelingskeuken
d Abteilungsküche *f*

648 FOOD DISTRIBUTION;
MEALS DISTRIBUTION
f distribution *f* de la nourriture;
distribution *f* des aliments;
distribution *f* des repas
e distribución *f* de alimentos;
distribución *f* de las comidas
i distribuzione *f* dei pasti
n voedseldistributie;
voedselverdeling;
maaltijddistributie;
maaltijdverdeling
d Speisenverteilung *f*;
Mahlzeitverteilung *f*

649 FOOD HYGIENE;
NUTRITIONAL HYGIENE
f hygiène *f* de l'alimentation

e higiene *f* de alimentos
i igiene *f* alimentare
n voedingshygiëne
d Lebensmittelhygiene *f*; Ernährungshygiene *f*

650 FOOD SERVICE; NUTRITION SERVICE
f service *m* de l'alimentation; service *m* de la nourriture
e servicio *m* de alimentos; servicio *m* de alimentación; servicio *m* de nutrición
i servizio *m* dell'alimentazione
n voedingsdienst
d Nahrungsdienst *m*

651 FORENSIC MEDICINE
f médecine *f* légale
e medicina *f* judicial
i medicina *f* legale
n gerechtelijke geneeskunde
d gerichtliche Medizin *f*

652 FULL TIME PHYSICIAN; FULL TIME PRACTITIONER
f médecin *m* à plein temps
e médico *m* a tiempo completo
i medico *m* a tempo pieno
n full time arts
d Full Time Arzt *m*

653 FULL TIME PRACTITIONER
see: FULL TIME PHYSICIAN

654 FUNCTIONAL REHABILITATION
f réadaptation *f* fonctionelle; révalidation *f* fonctionelle; réhabilitation *f* fonctionelle; rééducation *f* fonctionelle
e revalidación *f* funcional; rehabilitación *f* funcional; readaptación *f* funcional
i riabilitazione *f* funzionale; riadattamento *m* funzionale; rieducazione *f* funzionale
n functionele revalidatie; functionele reactivering
d funktionelle Rehabilitation *f*

655 FUNERAL PARLOUR
f chapelle *f* ardente
e capilla *f* ardiente
i camera *f* ardente
n rouwkamer
d Trauerkapelle *f*

G

656 GASTRO-ENTEROLOGIST
f gastro-entérologue *m*
e gastroenterólogo *m*
i gastroenterologo *m*
n gastro-enteroloog
d Gastroenterologe *m*

657 GASTRO-ENTEROLOGY
f gastro-entérologie *f*
e gastroenterología *f*
i gastroenterologia *f*
n gastro-enterologie
d Gastroenterologie *f*

658 GASTRO-ENTEROLOGY DEPARTMENT
f service *m* (département *m*) de gastro-entérologie
e servicio *m* (departamento *m*) de gastroenterología
i servizio *m* di gastroenterologia
n gastro-enterologische afdeling
d gastroenterologische Abteilung *f*

659 GASTRO-ENTEROLOGY UNIT
f unité *f* de gastro-entérologie
e unidad *f* de gastroenterología
i unità *f* di gastroenterologia
n gastro-enterologische eenheid
d gastroenterologische Station *f*

660 GASTROSCOPY
f gastroscopie *f*
e gastroscopia *f*
i gastroscopia *f*
n gastroscopie
d Gastroskopie *f*

661 GENERAL HOSPITAL
f hôpital *m* général;
établissement *m* hospitalier général;
établissement *m* d'hospitalisation général;
institution *f* hospitalière générale;
établissement *m* polyvalent
e hospital *m* general;
institución *f* hospitalaria general
i ospedale *m* generale;
stabilimento *m* ospedaliero generale
n algemeen ziekenhuis *n*
d allgemeines Krankenhaus *n*;
Allgemeinkrankenhaus *n*;
allgemeines Spital *n*;
Allgemeinspital *n*

662 GENERALIST
see: FAMILY DOCTOR

663 GENERAL MEDICAL CLINIC
f clinique *f* de médecine générale
e clínica *f* de medicina general
i clinica *f* medica generale
n kliniek voor algemene geneeskunde
d Klinik *f* für allgemeine Medizin

664 GENERAL MEDICINE
f médecine *f* générale
e medicina *f* general
i medicina *f* generale
n algemene geneeskunde
d allgemeine Medizin *f*;
Allgemeinmedizin *f*

665 GENERAL MEDICINE DEPARTMENT
f service *m* (département *m*) de médecine générale
e servicio *m* (departamento *m*) de medicina general
i divisione *f* di medicina generale
n afdeling voor algemene geneeskunde
d Abteilung *f* für allgemeine Medizin

666 GENERAL NURSING STUDENT;
GENERAL STUDENT NURSE
f élève-infirmière *f* générale;
apprentie-infirmière *f* générale
e enfermera *f* alumna general;
alumna *f* de enfermera general
i allieva *f* infermiera generale
n A-leerling-verpleegkundige;
A-leerling-verplegende;
A-leerling-verpleegster
d allgemeine Pflegeschülerin *f*;
allgemeine Krankenpflegeschülerin *f*

667 GENERAL PRACTICE
f cabinet *m* de médecine générale
e práctica *f* general de la medicina
i gabinetto *m* di medicina generale
n huisartsenpraktijk
d Allgemeinpraxis *f*

668 GENERAL PRACTITIONER
see: FAMILY DOCTOR

669 GENERAL STUDENT NURSE
see: GENERAL NURSING STUDENT

670 GENERAL SURGEON
f chirurgien *m* général
e cirujano *m* general
i chirurgo *m* generale
n algemeen chirurg
d allgemeiner Chirurg *m*

671 GENERAL SURGERY
f chirurgie *f* générale
e cirugía *f* general
i chirurgia *f* generale
n algemene chirurgie
d allgemeine Chirurgie *f*

672 GENERAL SURGERY DEPARTMENT
f service *m* (département *m*) de chirurgie générale
e servicio *m* (departamento *m*) de cirugía general
i divisione *f* di chirurgia generale
n algemene chirurgische afdeling
d Abteilung *f* für allgemeine Chirurgie

673 GERIATRIC CARE
f soins *mpl* gériatriques
e cuidado *m* geriátrico;
atención *f* (asistencia *f*) geriátrica
i assistenza *f* agli anziani
n geriatrische zorg
d geriatrische Versorgung *f*

674 GERIATRIC CENTRE (CENTER)
f centre *m* gériatrique;
centre *m* de gériatrie
e centro *m* geriátrico;
centro *m* de geriatría
i centro *m* di cura per gli anziani
n geriatrisch centrum *n*;
bejaardencentrum *n*
d geriatrisches Zentrum *n*

675 GERIATRIC CLINIC
f clinique *f* gériatrique;
clinique *f* de gériatrie
e clínica *f* geriátrica;
clínica *f* de geriatría
i clinica *f* geriatrica
n geriatrische kliniek
d geriatrische Klinik *f*

676 GERIATRIC DAY HOSPITAL
f hôpital *m* de jour gériatrique;
hôpital *m* de jour de gériatrie
e hospital *m* diurno geriátrico;
hospital *m* diurno de geriatría;
hospital *m* de día geriátrico;
hospital *m* de día de geriatría
i ospedale *m* geriatrico diurno
n geriatrisch dagziekenhuis *n*
d geriatrisches Tag(es)krankenhaus *n*;
geriatrisches Tagesspital *n*

677 GERIATRIC DEPARTMENT
f service *m* (département *m*) gériatrique;
service *m* (département *m*) de gériatrie
e servicio *m* (departamento *m*) geriátrico;
servicio *m* (departamento *m*) de geriatría
i divisione *f* di geriatria
n geriatrische afdeling;
afdeling voor bejaarden
d geriatrische Abteilung *f*;
Abteilung *f* für Alterspatienten

678 GERIATRIC HOME;
HOME FOR AGED PEOPLE;
HOME FOR OLD PEOPLE:
HOME FOR THE AGED;
OLD AGE HOME;
OLD PEOPLE HOME;
RESORT FOR THE AGED
f home *m* pour personnes âgées;
établissement *m* pour personnes âgées;
foyer *m* pour personnes âgées;
centre *m* pour personnes âgées;
maison *f* de vieillards;
asile *m* de vieillards
e asilo *m* para ancianos;
hogar *m* para ancianos;
hospicio *m* para ancianos
i casa *f* di riposo per anziani;
ospizio *m* per vecchi
n bejaardentehuis *n*;
tehuis voor bejaarden *n*;
bejaardenoord *n*
d Altenheim *n*;
Altersheim *n*;
Betagtenheim *n*

679 GERIATRIC HOSPITAL
f hôpital *m* gériatrique;
hôpital *m* de gériatrie
e hospital *m* geriátrico;
hospital *m* de geriatría
i ospedale *m* geriatrico
n ziekenhuis *n* voor bejaarden
d geriatrisches Krankenhaus *n*;
Alterskrankenhaus *n*

680 GERIATRIC NURSE
f infirmière *f* gériatrique
e enfermera *f* geriátrica
i infermiera *f* di geriatria
n bejaardenverzorgster
d Altenpflegerin *f*;
Pflegerin *f* für Betagte

681 GERIATRIC NURSING
f soins *mpl* infirmiers gériatriques
e enfermería *f* geriátrica;
cuidado *m* enfermero geriátrico;
atención *f* (asistencia *f*) enfermera geriátrica
i cure *fpl* infermieristiche geriatriche;
assistenza *f* infermieristica agli anziani
n geriatrische verpleging
d Altenpflege *f*

682 GERIATRIC NURSING HOME
f établissement *m* de soins gériatriques
e casa *f* de salud geriátrica
i ospedale *m* geriatrico
n verpleeghuis *n* voor bejaarden
d Altenpflegeheim *n*

683 GERIATRIC PATIENT
f malade *m* (patient *m*) gériatrique
e paciente *m* (enfermo *m*) geriátrico
i malato *m* geriatrico
n geriatrische patiënt
d Alterspatient *m*;
Alterskranker *m*;
geriatrischer Patient *m*

684 GERIATRICS
f gériatrie *f*
e geriatría *f*
i geriatria *f*
n geriatrie
d Geriatrie *f*

685 GERIATRIC UNIT
f unité *f* gériatrique;
unité *f* de gériatrie
e unidad *f* geriátrica;
unidad *f* de geriatría
i unità *f* di geriatria
n geriatrische eenheid
d geriatrische Station *f*

686 GERONTOLOGIST
f gérontologiste *m*;
gérontologue *m*
e gerontólogo *m*
i gerontologo *m*
n gerontoloog
d Gerontologe *m*

687 GERONTOLOGY
f gérontologie *f*
e gerontología *f*
i gerontologia *f*
n gerontologie
d Gerontologie *f*

688 GRADUATED CARE
f soins *mpl* gradués

e cuidado *m* graduado;
atención *f* graduada
i cure *fpl* graduate;
cure *fpl* per gradi
n graduele zorg
d graduelle Pflege *f*

689 GRADUATED TREATMENT
f traitement *m* gradué
e tratamiento *m* graduado
i trattamento *m* graduato;
trattamento *m* per gradi
n graduele behandeling
d graduelle Behandlung *f*

690 GRADUATE NURSE
see: DIPLOMA NURSE

691 GROUP MEDICINE
f médecine *f* de groupe
e medicina *f* de grupo
i medicina *f* di gruppo
n groepsgeneeskunde
d Gruppenmedizin *f*

692 GROUP NURSING;
GROUP NURSING CARE;
TEAM NURSING;
TEAM NURSING CARE
f soins *mpl* infirmiers de groupe
e enfermería *f* en equipo (grupo);
cuidado *m* enfermero en equipo (grupo);
atención *f* enfermera en equipo (grupo)
i cure *fpl* infermieristiche di gruppo
n groepsverpleging;
teamverpleging
d Gruppenpflege *f*

693 GROUP NURSING CARE
see: GROUP NURSING

694 GROUP PRACTICE
f cabinet *m* médical de groupe
e grupo *m* médico
i gabinetto *m* medico di gruppo;
gruppo *m* medico
n groepspraktijk
d Gruppenpraxis *f*

695 GROUP THERAP(EUT)IST
f thérapeute *m* de groupe
e terapeuta *m* de grupo
i terapeuta *m* (terapista *m*) di gruppo
n groepstherapeut
d Gruppentherapeut *m*

696 GROUP THERAPY
f thérapie *f* de groupe
e terapia *f* grupal;
terapia *f* de grupo
i terapia *f* di gruppo
n groepstherapie
d Gruppentherapie *f*

697 GYNECOLOGICAL CLINIC;
GYNECOLOGY CLINIC;
WOMEN'S CLINIC
f clinique *f* gynécologique;
clinique *f* de gynécologie
e clínica *f* ginecológica;
clínica *f* de ginecología
i clinica *f* ginecologica
n vrouwenkliniek;
gynecologische kliniek
d Frauenklinik *f*;
gynäkologische Klinik *f*

698 GYNECOLOGICAL DEPARTMENT;
GYNECOLOGY DEPARTMENT;
WOMEN'S DEPARTMENT
f service *m* (département *m*) gynécologique;
service *m* (département *m*) de gynécologie
e servicio *m* (departamento *m*) ginecológico;
servicio *m* (departamento *m*) de ginecología
i divisione *f* di ginecologia
n vrouwenafdeling;
gynecologische afdeling
d Frauenabteilung *f*;
gynäkologische Abteilung *f*

699 GYNECOLOGICAL HOSPITAL;
GYNECOLOGY HOSPITAL;
WOMEN'S HOSPITAL
f hôpital *m* gynécologique;
hôpital *m* de gynécologie
e hospital *m* ginecológico;
hospital *m* de ginecología
i ospedale *m* ginecologico
n vrouwenziekenhuis *n*;
gynecologisch ziekenhuis *n*
d Frauenkrankenhaus *n*;
gynäkologisches Krankenhaus *n*

700 GYNECOLOGICAL UNIT;
GYNECOLOGY UNIT;
WOMEN'S UNIT
f unité *f* gynécologique;
unité *f* de gynécologie
e unidad *f* ginecológica;
unidad *f* de ginecología
i unità *f* ginecologica
n vrouweneenheid;
gynecologische eenheid
d Frauenstation *f*;
gynäkologische Station *f*

701 GYNECOLOGIST
f gynécologue *m*;
gynécologiste *m*
e ginecólogo *m*
i ginecologo *m*
n gynecoloog;
vrouwenarts
d Gynäkologe *m*;
Frauenarzt *m*

702 GYNECOLOGY
f gynécologie *f*
e ginecología *f*
i ginecologia *f*
n gynecologie
d Gynäkologie *f*

703 GYNECOLOGY CLINIC
see: GYNECOLOGICAL CLINIC

704 GYNECOLOGY DEPARTMENT
see: GYNECOLOGICAL DEPARTMENT

705 GYNECOLOGY HOSPITAL
see: GYNECOLOGICAL HOSPITAL

706 GYNECOLOGY UNIT
see: GYNECOLOGICAL UNIT

H

707 HANDICAPPED CHILD CARE
f soins *mpl* aux enfants handicapés
e cuidado *m* (atención *f*) de los niños impedidos;
asistencia *f* a los niños impedidos
i cure *fpl* dell'infanzia handicappata
n zorg voor gehandicapte kinderen
d Fürsorge *f* für behinderte Kinder

708 HEAD NURSE
see: CHIEF NURSE

709 HEAD OF THE NURSING SERVICE;
MATRON
f infirmière-chef *f* de service
e jefe *f* de enfermeras
i responsabile *f* del servizio infermieristico
n hoofd *n* verplegingsdienst;
hoofd *n* verpleegkundige dienst
d Leiterin *f* des Pflegedienstes;
Oberin *f*

710 HEAD PHYSICIAN
see: CHIEF DOCTOR

711 HEAD SURGEON
f chirurgien *m* en chef
e cirujano *m* en jefe
i primario *m* di chirurgia
n hoofdchirurg
d Chef *m* Chirurgie

712 HEALTH
f santé *f*
e salud *f*
i salute *f*;
sanità *f*
n gezondheid
d Gesundheit *f*

713 HEALTH AUTHORITIES
f autorités *fpl* sanitaires;
autorités *fpl* de la santé
e autoridades *fpl* sanitarias;
autoridades *fpl* de salud
i autorità *fpl* sanitarie
n gezondheidsoverheden
d Gesundheitsbehörden *fpl*

714 HEALTH BUDGET
f budget *m* sanitaire;
budget *m* de la santé
e presupuesto *m* sanitario;
presupuesto *m* de salud
i budget *m* sanitario
n budget *n* voor gezondheidszorg
d Gesundheitsbudget *n*

715 HEALTH CARE
f soins *mpl* sanitaires;
soins *mpl* de santé
e cuidado *m* sanitario;
atención *f* (asistencia *f*) sanitaria;
cuidado *m* (atención *f*) de la salud
i assistenza *f* sanitaria
n gezondheidszorg
d Gesundheitsfürsorge *f*;
Gesundheitspflege *f*;
Krankenfürsorge *f*;
gesundheitliche Versorgung *f*

716 HEALTH CARE CENTRE (CENTER);
HEALTH CENTRE (CENTER)
f centre *m* sanitaire;
centre *m* de santé
e centro *m* sanitario;
centro *m* de salud
i centro *m* sanitario
n gezondheidscentrum *n*
d Gesundheitszentrum *n*

717 HEALTH CARE COSTS
f coûts *mpl* de soins sanitaires
e gastos *mpl* sanitarios;
gastos *mpl* de cuidado sanitario
i costi *mpl* dell' assistenza sanitaria
n kosten van gezondheidszorg
d Gesundheitsfürsorgekosten *pl*

718 HEALTH CARE DELIVERY
f dispensation *f* de services sanitaires;
dispensation *f* de services de santé
e prestación *f* sanitaria;
prestación *f* de servicios de salud
i servizi *mpl* sanitari
n gezondheidszorgverstrekking
d Gesundheitsfürsorgeleistung *f*

719 HEALTH CARE EXPENDITURES;
HEALTH CARE EXPENSES;
HEALTH EXPENDITURES;
HEALTH EXPENSES
f dépenses *fpl* sanitaires;
dépenses *fpl* de santé
e gastos *mpl* sanitarios;
gastos *mpl* de salud;
gastos *mpl* de sanidad
i spese *fpl* per i servizi sanitari
n uitgaven voor gezondheidszorg
d Gesundheitsfürsorgeausgaben *fpl*

720 HEALTH CARE EXPENSES
see: HEALTH CARE EXPENDITURES

721 HEALTH CARE FACILITIES;
HEALTH CARE SERVICES;
HEALTH FACILITIES;
HEALTH SERVICES
f services *mpl* sanitaires;
services *mpl* de santé
e servicios *mpl* sanitarios;
servicios *mpl* de salud;
servicios *mpl* de sanidad
i servizi *mpl* sanitari
n gezondheidsvoorzieningen;
gezondheidsdiensten
d Gesundheitsfürsorgedienste *mpl*

722 HEALTH CARE INSTITUTION;
HEALTH INSTITUTION;
SANITARY INSTITUTION
f établissement *m* sanitaire;

établissement *m* de santé;
institution *f* sanitaire;
institution *f* de santé
e institución *f* sanitaria;
institución *f* de salud;
instalación *f* sanitaria;
instalación *f* de salud
i istituto *m* sanitario;
stabilimento *m* sanitario
n instelling voor gezondheidszorg;
inrichting voor gezondheidszorg
d Gesundheits(pflege)einrichtung *f*;
Einrichtung *f* des Gesundheitswesens

723 HEALTH CARE INSURANCE;
HEALTH (COSTS) INSURANCE;
SICKNESS (COSTS) INSURANCE
f assurance-maladie *f*;
assurance *f* contre la maladie
e seguro *m* de enfermedad;
seguro *m* de salud
i assicurazione *f* malattia;
assicurazione *f* contro le malattie
n ziekte(kosten)verzekering
d Krankenversicherung *f*

724 HEALTH CARE MANAGEMENT;
HEALTH MANAGEMENT
f gestion *f* sanitaire;
gestion *f* de la santé
e gestión *f* sanitaria;
gestión *f* de salud
i gestione *f* sanitaria
n gezondheidszorgbeleid *n*
d Gesundheitsverwaltung *f*

725 HEALTH CARE MANPOWER;
HEALTH CARE PERSONNEL;
HEALTH CARE STAFF;
HEALTH MANPOWER;
HEALTH PERSONNEL;
HEALTH STAFF
f personnel *m* sanitaire;
personnel *m* de santé
e personal *m* sanitario;
personal *m* de salud;
personal *m* de sanidad
i personale *m* sanitario
n gezondheidspersoneel *n*
d Gesundheitspersonal *n*

726 HEALTH CARE ORGANIZATION;
HEALTH ORGANIZATION;
SANITARY ORGANIZATION
f organisation *f* sanitaire
e organización *f* sanitaria;
organización *f* de salud
i organizzazione *f* sanitaria
n organisatie van de gezondheidszorg;
gezondheidsorganisatie
d Gesundheitsorganisation *f*

727 HEALTH CARE PERSONNEL
see: HEALTH CARE MANPOWER

728 HEALTH CARE PLANNING;
HEALTH PLANNING;
SANITARY PLANNING
f planification *f* sanitaire
e planificación *f* sanitaria;
planificación *f* de salud;
planeamiento *m* sanitario;
planeamiento *m* de salud
i pianificazione *f* sanitaria
n gezondheidszorgplanning
d Gesundheitsfürsorgeplanung *f*

729 HEALTH CARE POLICY;
HEALTH POLICY
f politique *f* sanitaire;
politique *f* de santé
e política *f* sanitaria;
política *f* de salud
i politica *f* sanitaria
n gezondheidspolitiek
d Gesundheitspolitik *f*

730 HEALTH CARE PRIORITIES
f priorités *fpl* en matière de soins sanitaires
e prioridades *fpl* en cuidado sanitario
i priorità *fpl* nella assistenza sanitaria
n prioriteiten in de gezondheidszorg
d Gesundheitsfürsorgeprioritäten *fpl*

731 HEALTH CARE SERVICES
see: HEALTH CARE FACILITIES

732 HEALTH CARE STAFF
see: HEALTH CARE MANPOWER

733 HEALTH CARE STRUCTURE;
HEALTH STRUCTURE
f structure *f* sanitaire
e estructura *f* sanitaria
i struttura *f* sanitaria
n gezondheidszorgstructuur;
structuur van de gezondheidszorg
d Struktur *f* des Gesundheitswesens

734 HEALTH CARE SYSTEM;
HEALTH SYSTEM
f système *m* sanitaire;
système *m* de santé
e sistema *m* sanitario;
sistema *m* de salud
i sistema *m* sanitario
n gezondheidszorgsysteem *n*
d System *n* des Gesundheitswesens

735 HEALTH CARE TEAM;
HEALTH TEAM
f équipe *f* sanitaire;
équipe *f* de santé
e equipo *m* sanitario
i équipe *f* sanitaria;
équipe *f* d'igiene
n verzorgingsteam *n*
d Gesundheitsteam *n*

736 HEALTH CARE UTILIZATION
f utilisation *f* des services sanitaires
e utilización *f* de servicios sanitarios
i utilizzazione *f* dei servizi sanitari
n gebruik *n* van gezondheidszorgdiensten
d Ausnutzung *f* von Gesundheitsdiensten

737 HEALTH CENTRE (CENTER)
see: HEALTH CARE CENTRE (CENTER)

738 HEALTH CONDITION;
HEALTH STATUS
f état *m* sanitaire;
état *m* de santé;
conditions *fpl* sanitaires;

conditions *fpl* hygiéniques
e estado *m* de salud
i stato *m* di salute;
situazione *f* sanitaria;
condizioni *fpl* igienico-sanitarie
n gezondheidstoestand
d Gesundheitszustand *m*

739 HEALTH CONTROL
f contrôle *m* de santé
e control *m* sanitario
i controllo *m* sanitario
n gezondheidscontrole
d Gesundheitsüberwachung *f*

740 HEALTH COSTS INSURANCE
see: HEALTH CARE INSURANCE

741 HEALTH ECOLOGY
f écologie *f* sanitaire;
écologie *f* de santé
e ecología *f* sanitaria;
ecología *f* de salud
i ecologia *f* sanitaria
n gezondheidsecologie
d Gesundheitsekologie *f*

742 HEALTH ECONOMICS;
SANITARY ECONOMICS
f économie *f* sanitaire;
économie *f* de santé
e economía *f* sanitaria;
economía *f* de salud
i economia *f* sanitaria
n gezondheidseconomie
d Gesundheitswirtschaft *f*

743 HEALTH ECONOMIST;
SANITARY ECONOMIST
f économe *m* de santé
e economista *m* de salud
i economista *m* specializzato in problemi sanitari
n gezondheidseconoom
d Gesundheitswirtschaftler *m*;
Gesundheitsökonom *m*

744 HEALTH EDUCATION;
SANITARY EDUCATION
f éducation *f* sanitaire;
éducation *f* pour la santé
e educación *f* sanitaria;
educación *f* de la salud;
educación *f* de la higiene
i educazione *f* sanitaria
n gezondheidsopvoeding
d Gesundheitserziehung *f*

745 HEALTH EXPENDITURES
see: HEALTH CARE EXPENDITURES

746 HEALTH EXPENSES
see: HEALTH CARE EXPENDITURES

747 HEALTH FACILITIES
see: HEALTH CARE FACILITIES

748 HEALTH FACILITIES ADMINISTRATION
f administration *f* de services sanitaires
e administración *f* de servicios sanitarios
i amministrazione *f* dei servizi sanitari
n administratie van gezondheidsvoorzieningen
d Verwaltung *f* von Gesundheitsfürsorgediensten

749 HEALTH FACILITIES PLANNING
f planification *f* de services sanitaires
e planificación *f* de servicios sanitarios;
planeamiento *m* de servicios sanitarios
i pianificazione *f* dei servizi sanitari
n planning van gezondheidsvoorzieningen
d Planung *f* von Gesundheitsfürsorgediensten

750 HEALTH INFORMATION
f information *f* sanitaire
e información *f* sanitaria
i informazione *f* sanitaria
n gezondheidsvoorlichting
d Gesundheitsaufklärung *f*

751 HEALTH INSTITUTION
see: HEALTH CARE INSTITUTION

752 HEALTH INSURANCE
see: HEALTH CARE INSURANCE

753 HEALTH INSURANCE COMPANY
f compagnie *f* d'assurance-maladie
e compañía *f* de seguro de enfermedad
i compagnia *f* di assicurazione malattia
n ziekte(kosten)verzekeraar;
ziekte(kosten)verzekeringsmaatschappij
d Krankenversicherungsgesellschaft *f*

754 HEALTH INSURANCE FUND;
SICK-FUND
f caisse *f* d'assurance-maladie;
caisse *f* (de) maladie
e caja *f* de seguro de enfermedad;
caja *f* de enfermedad
i cassa-mutua *f*
n ziekenfonds *n*
d Krankenkasse *f*

755 HEALTH INSURANCE LEGISLATION
f législation *f* en matière d'assurance-maladie
e legislación *f* sobre el seguro de enfermedad
i legislazione *f* in materia di assicurazione malattia
n wetgeving op de ziekte(kosten)verzekering
d Gesetzgebung *f* für Krankenversicherung

756 HEALTH INSURANCE SYSTEM
f système *m* d'assurance-maladie
e sistema *m* de seguro de enfermedad
i sistema *m* di assicurazione malattia
n ziekte(kosten)verzekeringssysteem *n*
d Krankenversicherungswesen *n*

757 HEALTH LEGISLATION
f législation *f* sanitaire
e legislación *f* sanitaria
i legislazione *f* sanitaria
n gezondheidswetgeving
d Gesundheitsgesetzgebung *f*

758 HEALTH MANAGEMENT
see: HEALTH CARE MANAGEMENT

759 HEALTH MANPOWER
see: HEALTH CARE MANPOWER

760 HEALTH MANPOWER PLANNING
f planification *f* de personnel sanitaire
e planificación *f* de personal sanitario;
planeamiento *m* de personal sanitario
i pianificazione *f* del personale sanitario
n planning van gezondheidspersoneel
d Planung *f* von Gesundheitspersonal

761 HEALTH ORGANIZATION
see: HEALTH CARE ORGANIZATION

762 HEALTH PERSONNEL
see: HEALTH CARE MANPOWER

763 HEALTH PLANNING
see: HEALTH CARE PLANNING

764 HEALTH POLICY
see: HEALTH CARE POLICY

765 HEALTH PROFESSION
f profession *f* sanitaire
e profesión *f* sanitaria
i professione *f* sanitaria
n beroep *n* in de gezondheidszorg
d Gesundheitsberuf *m*;
Heilberuf *m*

766 HEALTH PROTECTION;
SANITARY PROTECTION
f protection *f* sanitaire;
protection *f* de la santé
e protección *f* sanitaria;
protección *f* de la salud
i protezione *f* sanitaria
n gezondheidsbescherming
d Gesundheitsschutz *m*

767 HEALTH REFORM;
SANITARY REFORM
f réforme *f* sanitaire
e reforma *f* sanitaria
i riforma *f* sanitaria
n hervorming van de gezondheidszorg
d Gesundheitsfürsorgereform *f*

768 HEALTH REGION
f région *f* sanitaire
e región *f* sanitaria
i regione *f* sanitaria
n gezondheidsregio
d Gesundheitsregion *f*

769 HEALTH RESEARCH
f recherche *f* sanitaire
e investigación *f* sanitaria
i ricerca *f* sanitaria
n gezondheidsonderzoek *n*
d Gesundheitsforschung *f*

770 HEALTH RISK
f risques *mpl* de la santé
e riesgo *m* de la salud
i rischio *m* di malattia
n gezondheidsrisico *n*
d Gesundheitsrisiko *n*

771 HEALTH SCHOOL
f école *f* de santé
e escuela *f* de salud
i scuola *f* di sanità
n gezondheidsschool
d Schule *f* für Gesundheit

772 HEALTH SCIENCE
f science *f* sanitaire;
science *f* de la santé
e ciencia *f* sanitaria;
ciencia *f* de la salud
i scienza *f* sanitaria
n gezondheidkunde
d Gesundheitswissenschaft *f*

773 HEALTH SCIENCE CENTRE (CENTER)
f centre *m* sanitaire scientifique
e centro *m* de ciencias sanitarias
i centro *m* sanitario scientifico
n centrum *n* voor gezondheidkunde
d Zentrum *n* für Gesundheitswissenschaft

774 HEALTH SERVICES
see: HEALTH CARE FACILITIES

775 HEALTH STAFF
see: HEALTH CARE MANPOWER

776 HEALTH STATISTICS
f statistique *f* sanitaire
e estadística *f* sanitaria
i statistica *f* sanitaria
n gezondheidsstatistiek
d Gesundheitsstatistik *f*

777 HEALTH STATUS
see: HEALTH CONDITION

778 HEALTH STRUCTURE
see: HEALTH CARE STRUCTURE

779 HEALTH SYSTEM
see: HEALTH CARE SYSTEM

780 HEALTH TEAM
see: HEALTH CARE TEAM

781 HEALTH TRANSPORT(ATION);
PATIENT TRANSPORT(ATION)
f transport *m* sanitaire;
transport *m* des malades
e transporte *m* sanitario;
transporte *m* de enfermos
i trasporto *m* sanitario;
trasporto *m* dei malati
n ziekenvervoer *n*
d Krankentransport *m*;
Patiententransport *m*

782 HEALTH WORKER
f agent *m* sanitaire;
technicien *m* de la santé
e trabajador *m* de salud;
técnico *m* de sanidad
i tecnico *m* sanitario
n gezondheidswerker;
werker in de gezondheidszorg
d Gesundheitstechniker *m*

783 HEART CENTRE (CENTER)
see: CARDIOLOGY CENTRE (CENTER)

784 HEART DISEASE
f maladie *f* du coeur
e enfermedad *f* cardíaca;
enfermedad *f* del corazón
i malattia *f* di cuore
n hartziekte
d Herzkrankheit *f*

785 HEART EXAMINATION
f examen *m* cardiaque;
examen *m* du cœur
e examen *m* cardíaco;

examen *m* del corazón
i esame *m* del cuore
n hartonderzoek *n*
d Herzuntersuchung *f*

786 HEART MASSAGE
f massage *m* cardiaque;
massage *m* du cœur
e masage *m* cardíaco;
masage *m* del corazón
i massaggio *m* cardiaco
n hartmassage
d Herzmassage *f*

787 HEART MONITORING
f surveillance *f* cardiaque;
surveillance *f* du cœur
e vigilancia *f* cardíaca;
vigilancia *f* del corazón
i sorveglianza *f* cardiaca
n hartbewaking
d Herzüberwachung *f*

788 HEART REHABILITATION
f révalidation *f* cardiaque;
révalidation *f* du cœur
e revalidación *f* cardíaca;
revalidación *f* del corazón
i riabilitazione *f* cardiaca
n hartrevalidatie
d Herzrehabilitation *f*

789 HEART SURGERY
f chirurgie *f* cardiaque;
chirurgie *f* du cœur
e cirugía *f* cardíaca;
cirugía *f* del corazón
i cardiochirurgia *f*;
chirurgia *f* del cuore
n hartchirurgie
d Herzchirurgie *f*

790 HELIOTHERAPY
f héliothérapie *f*
e helioterapia *f*
i elioterapia *f*
n heliotherapie
d Heliotherapie *f*

791 HEMATOLOGIST
f hématologue *m*;
hématologiste *m*
e hematólogo *m*
i ematologo *m*
n hematoloog
d Hämatologe *m*

792 HEMATOLOGY
f hématologie *f*
e hematología *f*
i ematologia *f*
n hematologie
d Hämatologie *f*

793 HEMATOLOGY CLINIC
f clinique *f* hématologique;
clinique *f* d'hématologie
e clínica *f* hematológica;
clínica *f* de hematología
i clinica *f* ematologica
n hematologische kliniek
d hämatologische Klinik *f*

794 HEMATOLOGY DEPARTMENT
f service *m* (département *m*) hématologique;
service *m* (département *m*) d'hématologie
e servicio *m* (departamento *m*) hematológico;
servicio *m* (departamento *m*) de hematología
i servizio *m* ematologico
n hematologische afdeling
d hämatologische Abteilung *f*

795 HEMATOLOGY LABORATORY
f laboratoire *m* hématologique;
laboratoire *m* d'hématologie
e laboratorio *m* hematológico;
laboratorio *m* de hematología
i laboratorio *m* ematologico
n hematologisch laboratorium *n*
d hämatologisches Laboratorium *n*;
Laboratorium *n* für Hämatologie

796 HEMATOLOGY UNIT
f unité *f* hématologique;
unité *f* d'hématologie
e unidad *f* hematológica;
unidad *f* de hematología
i unità *f* ematologica
n hematologische eenheid
d hämatologische Station *f*

797 HEMODIALYSIS
f hémodialyse *f*
e hemodiálisis *f*
i emodialisi *f*
n hemodialyse
d Hämodialyse *f*

798 HEMOPHILIA
f hémophilie *f*
e hemofilia *f*
i emofilia *f*
n hemofilie
d Hämophilie *f*

799 HIGH CARE;
INTENSIVE CARE;
MAXIMUM CARE
f soins *mpl* intensifs;
soins *mpl* maxima
e cuidado *m* intensivo;
atención *f* intensiva;
cuidado *m* máximo;
atención *f* máxima
i cure *fpl* intensive
n intensieve zorg
d Intensivpflege *f*;
Maximalversorgung *f*

800 HIGH CARE DEPARTMENT;
INTENSIVE CARE DEPARTMENT
f service *m* (département *m*) de soins intensifs
e servicio *m* (departamento *m*) de cuidado intensivo
i servizio *m* di cure intensive
n afdeling voor intensieve zorg
d Intensivpflegeabteilung *f*

801 HIGH CARE UNIT;
INTENSIVE CARE UNIT
f unité *f* de soins intensifs
e unidad *f* de cuidado intensivo
i unità *f* di cure intensive
n eenheid voor intensieve zorg;
intensieve verpleegeenheid;
eenheid voor intensieve bewaking

d Intensiv(pflege)station *f*;
Intensivüberwachungsstation *f*

802 HIGH-LOW BED
f lit *m* réglable en hauteur
e cama *f* regulable en altura
i letto *m* regolabile in altezza
n hoog-laagbed *n*
d Niveaubett *n*

803 HISTORY OF MEDICINE;
MEDICAL HISTORY
f histoire *f* de la médecine
e historia *f* de la medicina
i storia *f* della medicina
n geschiedenis van de geneeskunde
d Geschichte *f* der Medizin

804 HISTORY OF NURSING;
NURSING HISTORY
f histoire *f* des soins infirmiers
e historia *f* de la enfermería
i storia *f* dell'assistenza infermieristica
n geschiedenis van de verpleging
d Geschichte *f* der Krankenpflege

805 HOME CARE
see: DOMICILIARY CARE

806 HOME DIALYSIS
f dialyse *f* à domicile
e diálisis *f* a domicilio
i dialisi *f* a domicilio
n thuisdialyse
d Dialyse *f* zu Hause

807 HOME FOR AGED PEOPLE
see: GERIATRIC HOME

808 HOME FOR LONG STAY PATIENTS
see: CHRONIC CARE INSTITUTION

809 HOME FOR OLD PEOPLE
see: GERIATRIC HOME

810 HOME FOR THE AGED
see: GERIATRIC HOME

811 HOME FOR TREATMENT OF ALCOHOLICS
f hôpital *m* de désintoxication
e sanatorio *m* de bebedores
i ospedale *m* di disintossicazione
n kliniek voor alcoholverslaafden
d Trinkerheilstätte *f*

812 HOME HEALTH CARE
see: DOMICILIARY CARE

813 HOME HELP
f aide *f* familiale;
auxiliaire *f* familiale;
travailleuse *f* familiale
e trabajadora *f* social de familia
i ausiliaria *f* familiare;
assistente *f* familiare
n gezinshulp;
gezinsverzorgster
d Hausfrauenablöserin *f*

814 HOME HELP SERVICE
f service *m* d'aides familiales
e servicio *m* social familiar
i servizio *m* di assistenza familiare
n dienst voor gezinszorg
d Dienst *m* für Hauspflege

815 HOME HOSPITALIZATION;
HOSPITAL CARE AT HOME;
HOSPITAL HOME CARE
f hospitalisation *f* à domicile;
dispensation *f* à domicile de soins hospitaliers
e hospitalización *f* domiciliaria;
hospitalización *f* a domicilio
i assistenza *f* ospedaliera a domicilio
n thuisverpleging
d Hospitalisierung *f* zu Hause

816 HOME NURSING
see: DOMICILIARY NURSING

817 HOME NURSING ORGANIZATION
see: CROSS ASSOCIATION

818 HOSPITAL
f hôpital *m*;
établissement *m* hospitalier;
établissement *m* d'hospitalisation;
institution *f* hospitalière
e hospital *m*;
institución *f* hospitalaria
i ospedale *m*;
stabilimento *m* ospedaliero
n ziekenhuis *n*;
ziekeninrichting
d Krankenhaus *n*;
Spital *n*;
Krankenanstalt *f*

819 HOSPITAL ACCREDITATION
f reconnaissance *f* de l'hôpital
e reconocimiento *m* del hospital
i riconoscimento *m* dell'ospedale
n erkenning van het ziekenhuis
d Anerkennung *f* des Krankenhauses

820 HOSPITAL ADMINISTRATION
f administration *f* hospitalière
e administración *f* hospitalaria
i amministrazione *f* ospedaliera
n ziekenhuisadministratie
d Krankenhausverwaltung *f*

821 HOSPITAL ADMINISTRATIVE DIRECTOR;
HOSPITAL ADMINISTRATOR
f directeur *m* administratif hospitalier;
administrateur *m* hospitalier;
administrateur *m* d'hôpital;
administrateur *m* gestionnaire d'hôpital
e director *m* administrativo hospitalario;
administrador *m* hospitalario;
administrador *m* del hospital
i direttore *m* amministrativo ospedaliero
n economisch ziekenhuisdirecteur;
directeur-econoom van een ziekenhuis;
administratief directeur van een ziekenhuis
d Krankenhausverwaltungsleiter *m*;
Krankenhausverwaltungsdirektor *m*

822 HOSPITAL ADMINISTRATOR
see: HOSPITAL ADMINISTRATIVE DIRECTOR

823 HOSPITAL ARCHITECTURE
f architecture *f* hospitalière
e arquitectura *f* hospitalaria

i architettura *f* ospedaliera
n ziekenhuisarchitectuur
d Krankenhausarchitektur *f*

824 HOSPITAL ARCHIVES;
HOSPITAL FILES;
HOSPITAL RECORDS
f archives *fpl* hospitalières
e archivo *m* hospitalario
i archivi *mpl* ospedalieri
n ziekenhuisarchief *n*
d Krankenhausarchiv *n*

825 HOSPITAL ASSOCIATION
f association *f* hospitalière
e asociación *f* hospitalaria
i associazione *f* ospedaliera
n ziekenhuisvereniging
d Krankenhausgesellschaft *f*

826 HOSPITAL AUTOPSY
f autopsie *f* hospitalière
e autopsia *f* hospitalaria
i autopsia *f* ospedaliera
n ziekenhuisautopsie
d Krankenhausautopsie *f*

827 HOSPITAL BED
see: COT

828 HOSPITAL BOARD;
HOSPITAL BOARD OF MANAGEMENT;
HOSPITAL BOARD OF TRUSTEES
f conseil *m* d'administration hospitalier
e consejo *m* de administración hospitalario;
representantes *mpl* del hospital
i consiglio *m* d'amministrazione dell'ospedale
n ziekenhuisbestuur *n*
d Krankenhausvorstand *m*

829 HOSPITAL BOARD OF MANAGEMENT
see: HOSPITAL BOARD

830 HOSPITAL BOARD OF TRUSTEES
see: HOSPITAL BOARD

831 HOSPITAL BUDGET
f budget *m* hospitalier
e presupuesto *m* hospitalario
i bilancio *m* ospedaliero
n ziekenhuisbudget *n*
d Krankenhausbudget *n*

832 HOSPITAL BUILDING;
HOSPITAL CONSTRUCTION
f construction *f* hospitalière
e construcción *f* hospitalaria
i costruzione *f* ospedaliera
n ziekenhuisbouw
d Krankenhausbau *m*;
Spitalbau *m*

833 HOSPITAL BUILDING SYSTEM
f système *m* de construction hospitalière
e sistema *m* de construcción hospitalaria
i sistema *m* di costruzione ospedaliera
n ziekenhuisbouwsysteem *n*
d Krankenhausbausystem *n*;
Spitalbausystem *n*

834 HOSPITAL CANTEEN
f cantine *f* hospitalière
e cantina *f* hospitalaria
i mensa *f* riservata al personale ospedaliero
n ziekenhuiskantine
d Krankenhauskantine *f*

835 HOSPITAL CAPACITY
f capacité *f* hospitalière
e capacidad *f* hospitalaria
i capacità *f* ospedaliera
n ziekenhuiscapaciteit
d Krankenhauskapazität *f*

836 HOSPITAL CARE
f soins *mpl* hospitaliers;
assistance *f* hospitalière
e cuidado *m* hospitalario;
atención *f* (asistencia *f*) hospitalaria
i cure *fpl* ospedaliere;
assistenza *f* ospedaliera
n ziekenhuisverzorging;
ziekenhuisverpleging;
ziekenhuiszorg
d Krankenhauspflege *f*;
Krankenhausbetreuung *f*;
Krankenhausversorgung *f*

837 HOSPITAL CARE AT HOME
see: HOME HOSPITALIZATION

838 HOSPITAL CARE COST
see: COST OF HOSPITAL CARE

839 HOSPITAL CENTRE (CENTER)
f centre *m* hospitalier
e centro *m* hospitalario
i centro *m* ospedaliero
n ziekenhuiscentrum *n*
d Krankenhauszentrum *n*

840 HOSPITAL CLOTHES
f vêtements *mpl* hospitaliers
e vestidos *mpl* hospitalarios
i abbigliamento *m* ospedaliero
n ziekenhuiskleding
d Krankenhauskleidung *f*

841 HOSPITAL COMMISSION;
HOSPITAL COMMITTEE
f comité *m* hospitalier
e comisión *f* hospitalaria
i comitato *m* ospedaliero
n ziekenhuiscommissie
d Krankenhauskommission *f*;
Krankenhausausschuss *m*

842 HOSPITAL COMMITTEE
see: HOSPITAL COMMISSION

843 HOSPITAL CONSTRUCTION
see: HOSPITAL BUILDING

844 HOSPITAL CONSULTANT;
HOSPITAL COUNSELLOR
f conseiller *m* hospitalier;
consultant *m* hospitalier
e consejero *m* hospitalario
i consigliere *m* ospedaliero
n ziekenhuisconsulent
d Krankenhausberater *m*

845 HOSPITAL COST
see: COST OF HOSPITAL CARE

846 HOSPITAL COUNSELLOR
see: HOSPITAL CONSULTANT

847 HOSPITAL DAY
see: DAY OF CARE

848 HOSPITAL DAY CARE
f soins *mpl* hospitaliers de jour
e cuidado *m* hospitalario diurno
i cure *fpl* ospedaliere diurne
n ziekenhuis-dagverzorging
d Krankenhaustagesversorgung *f*

849 HOSPITAL DEATH RATE;
HOSPITAL MORTALITY
f mortalité *f* hospitalière
e mortalidad *f* hospitalaria
i mortalità *f* ospedaliera
n ziekenhuismortaliteit
d Krankenhausmortalität *f*

850 HOSPITAL DENTIST
f dentiste *m* hospitalier
e dentista *m* hospitalario;
odontólogo *m* hospitalario
i dentista *m* ospedaliero
n ziekenhuistandarts
d Krankenhauszahnarzt *m*

851 HOSPITAL DEPARTMENT
f service *m* (département *m*) hospitalier
e servicio *m* (departamento *m*) hospitalario
i servizio *m* ospedaliero
n ziekenhuisafdeling
d Krankenhausabteilung *f*

852 HOSPITAL DIET
f régime *m* hospitalier
e dieta *f* hospitalaria
i regime *m* ospedaliero
n ziekenhuisdieet *n*
d Krankenhausdiät *n*

853 HOSPITAL DIETETICS
f diététique *f* hospitalière
e dietética *f* hospitalaria
i dietetica *f* ospedaliera
n ziekenhuisdiëtetiek
d Krankenhausdiätetik *f*

854 HOSPITAL DIRECTION;
HOSPITAL DIRECTORATE
f direction *f* hospitalière
e dirección *f* hospitalaria
i direzione *f* ospedaliera
n ziekenhuisdirectie;
ziekenhuisdirectorium *n*
d Krankenhausdirektion *f*;
Krankenhausdirektorium *n*

855 HOSPITAL DIRECTOR;
HOSPITAL MANAGER
f directeur *m* hospitalier
e director *m* hospitalario
i direttore *m* ospedaliero
n ziekenhuisdirecteur
d Krankenhausdirektor *m*;
Krankenhausleiter *m*

856 HOSPITAL DIRECTORATE
see: HOSPITAL DIRECTION

857 HOSPITAL DOCTOR;
HOSPITAL PHYSICIAN
f médecin *m* hospitalier
e médico *m* hospitalario;
doctor *m* hospitalario
i medico *m* ospedaliero
n ziekenhuisarts
d Krankenhausarzt *m*;
Spitalarzt *m*

858 HOSPITAL ECONOMICS
f économie *f* hospitalière
e economía *f* hospitalaria
i economia *f* ospedaliera
n ziekenhuiseconomie
d Krankenhauswirtschaft *f*

859 HOSPITAL EMPLOYEE
f agent *m* hospitalier
e empleado *m* hospitalario
i agente *m* ospedaliero
n ziekenhuiswerker
d Krankenhausangestellter *m*

860 HOSPITAL ENGINEER
f ingénieur *m* hospitalier
e ingeniero *m* hospitalario
i ingegnere *m* ospedaliero
n ziekenhuisingenieur
d Krankenhaus(betriebs)ingenieur *m*

861 HOSPITAL ENVIRONMENT
f milieu *m* hospitalier
e ambiente *m* hospitalario
i ambiente *m* ospedaliero
n ziekenhuismilieu *n*
d Krankenhausbereich *m*

862 HOSPITAL EQUIPMENT
f équipement *m* hospitalier
e equipo *m* hospitalario
i equipaggiamento *m* ospedaliero
n ziekenhuisuitrusting
d Krankenhausanlagen *fpl*

863 HOSPITAL FACILITIES;
HOSPITAL SERVICES
f armement *m* hospitalier;
services *mpl* hospitaliers
e servicios *mpl* hospitalarios;
red *f* hospitalaria;
instalaciones *fpl* hospitalarias
i servizi *mpl* ospedalieri
n ziekenhuisvoorzieningen;
ziekenhuiswezen *n*
d Krankenhauswesen *n*;
Spitalwesen *n*

864 HOSPITAL FEE;
HOSPITAL TARIFF
f tarif *m* hospitalier
e tarifa *f* hospitalaria
i tariffa *f* ospedaliera;
retta *f* di degenza
n ziekenhuistarief *n*
d Krankenhaustarif *m*

865 HOSPITAL FEE SETTING;
HOSPITAL TARIFF SETTING

f tarification *f* hospitalière
e fijación *f* de las tarifas hospitalarias
i determinazione *f* delle tariffe ospedaliere
n ziekenhuistarifering
d Krankenhaustarifsetzung *f*

866 HOSPITAL FILES
see: HOSPITAL ARCHIVES

867 HOSPITAL FINANCIAL MANAGEMENT
f gestion *f* financière hospitalière
e gestión *f* financiera hospitalaria
i gestione *f* finanziaria ospedaliera
n financieel beleid *n* van het ziekenhuis
d Krankenhausgeldgebarung *f*

868 HOSPITAL FINANCING
f financement *m* hospitalier
e financiación *f* hospitalaria
i finanziamento *m* ospedaliero
n ziekenhuisfinanciering
d Krankenhausfinanzierung *f*

869 HOSPITAL FOOD
f alimentation *f* hospitalière
e alimentación *f* hospitalaria
i alimentazione *f*ospedaliera
n ziekenhuisvoeding
d Krankenhausnahrung *f*

870 HOSPITAL (INSTITUTION) FOR MENTALLY DEFECTIVE;
HOSPITAL (INSTITUTION) FOR MENTALLY DEFICIENT;
HOSPITAL (INSTITUTION) FOR MENTALLY HANDICAPPED;
HOSPITAL (INSTITUTION) FOR MENTALLY RETARDED;
HOSPITAL (INSTITUTION) FOR MENTALLY SUBNORMAL
f établissement *m* (hôpital *m*) pour débiles mentaux (déficients mentaux, handicapés mentaux, retardés mentaux)
e hospital *m* (institución *f*) para débiles mentales (atrasados mentales, retardados mentales, disminuidos mentales)
i ospedale *m* per deficienti mentali (handicappati mentali)
n zwakzinnigeninrichting;
inrichting voor geestelijk gehandicapten
d Anstalt *f* für Schwachsinnige (Geistesschwache, Geistesbehinderte, geistig Behinderte)

871 HOSPITAL FOR MENTALLY DEFICIENT
see: HOSPITAL FOR MENTALLY DEFECTIVE

872 HOSPITAL FOR MENTALLY HANDICAPPED
see: HOSPITAL FOR MENTALLY DEFECTIVE

873 HOSPITAL FOR MENTALLY RETARDED
see: HOSPITAL FOR MENTALLY DEFECTIVE

874 HOSPITAL FOR MENTALLY SUBNORMAL
see: HOSPITAL FOR MENTALLY DEFECTIVE

875 HOSPITAL FURNITURE
f mobilier *m* hospitalier
e mueblaje *m* hospitalario
i mobili *mpl* per ospedali
n ziekenhuismeubilair *n*
d Krankenhausmobiliar *n*;
Krankenhausmobilien *pl*

876 HOSPITAL HOME CARE
see: HOME HOSPITALIZATION

877 HOSPITAL HYGIENE
f hygiène *f* hospitalière
e higiene *f* hospitalaria
i igiene *f* ospedaliera
n ziekenhuishygiëne
d Krankenhaushygiene *f*

878 HOSPITAL INFECTION
f infection *f* hospitalière
e infección *f* hospitalaria
i infezione *f* ospedaliera
n ziekenhuisinfectie;
hospitalisme *n*
d Krankenhausinfektion *f*;
Hospitalinfektion *f*;
Hospitalismus *m*

879 HOSPITAL INFORMATION SYSTEM
f système *m* d'information hospitalière
e sistema *m* de información hospitalaria
i informatica *f* ospedaliera
n ziekenhuis-informatiesysteem *n*
d Krankenhausinformationssystem *n*

880 HOSPITAL INPATIENT
see: BED PATIENT

881 HOSPITAL INSTITUTE
f institut *m* hospitalier
e instituto *m* hospitalario
i istituto *m* ospedaliero
n ziekenhuisinstituut *n*
d Krankenhausinstitut *n*

882 HOSPITAL INSURANCE;
HOSPITALIZATION INSURANCE
f assurance-hospitalisation *f*;
assurance *f* hospitalière
e seguro *m* de hospitalización;
seguro *m* de hospital
i assicurazione *f* per il ricovero in ospedale
n ziekenhuisverzekering
d Krankenhausversicherung *f*

883 HOSPITAL IN THE TROPICS
f hôpital *m* des tropiques
e hospital *m* de los trópicos
i ospedale *m* tropicale
n tropenziekenhuis *n*
d Tropenkrankenhaus *n*

884 HOSPITALIZATION;
INPATIENT HOSPITALIZATION;
INSTITUTIONALIZATION
f hospitalisation *f*
e hospitalización *f*
i ospedalizzazione *f*
n hospitalisatie
d Krankenhauseinweisung *f*

885 HOSPITALIZATION COST
see: COST OF HOSPITAL CARE

886 HOSPITALIZATION INSURANCE
see: HOSPITAL INSURANCE

887 HOSPITALIZATION LENGTH
see: DURATION OF HOSPITALIZATION

888 HOSPITALIZATION TIME
see: DURATION OF HOSPITALIZATION

889 HOSPITALIZED PATIENT
see: BED PATIENT

890 HOSPITAL JOURNAL;
HOSPITAL PERIODICAL
f revue *f* hospitalière
e revista *f* hospitalaria
i rivista *f* ospedaliera
n ziekenhuistijdschrift *n*
d Krankenhauszeitschrift *f*

891 HOSPITAL KITCHEN
f cuisine *f* hospitalière
e cocina *f* hospitalaria
i cucina *f* ospedaliera
n ziekenhuiskeuken
d Krankenhausküche *f*

892 HOSPITAL LABORATORY
f laboratoire *m* hospitalier
e laboratorio *m* hospitalario
i laboratorio *m* ospedaliero
n ziekenhuislaboratorium *n*
d Krankenhauslaboratorium *n*

893 HOSPITAL LAUNDRY
f blanchisserie *f* hospitalière;
buanderie *f* hospitalière
e lavadero *m* hospitalario
i lavanderia *f* ospedaliera
n ziekenhuiswasserij
d Krankenhauswäscherei *f*

894 HOSPITAL LAW
f loi *f* hospitalière
e ley *f* hospitalaria
i legge *f* ospedaliera
n ziekenhuiswet
d Krankenhausgesetz *n*;
Spitalgesetz *n*

895 HOSPITAL LEGISLATION
f législation *f* hospitalière
e legislación *f* hospitalaria
i legislazione *f* ospedaliera
n ziekenhuiswetgeving
d Krankenhausgesetzgebung *f*

896 HOSPITAL LIABILITY;
HOSPITAL RESPONSIBILITY
f responsabilité *f* hospitalière
e responsabilidad *f* hospitalaria
i responsabilità *f* ospedaliera
n ziekenhuisaansprakelijkheid;
ziekenhuisverantwoordelijkheid
d Krankenhaushaftpflicht *f*

897 HOSPITAL LIBRARY
f bibliothèque *f* hospitalière
e biblioteca *f* hospitalaria
i biblioteca *f* ospedaliera
n ziekenhuisbibliotheek
d Krankenhausbibliothek *f*;
Krankenhausbücherei *f*

898 HOSPITAL LITERATURE
f littérature *f* hospitalière
e literatura *f* hospitalaria
i letteratura *f* ospedaliera
n ziekenhuisliteratuur
d Krankenhausliteratur *f*

899 HOSPITAL LOAN
f émission *f* hospitalière
e empréstito *m* hospitalario
i emissione *f* ospedaliera
n ziekenhuislening
d Krankenhausanleihe *f*

900 HOSPITAL MANAGEMENT
f gestion *f* hospitalière
e gestión *f* hospitalaria
i gestione *f* ospedaliera
n ziekenhuisbeleid *n*
d Krankenhausleitung *f*

901 HOSPITAL MANAGER
see: HOSPITAL DIRECTOR

902 HOSPITAL MANPOWER;
HOSPITAL PERSONNEL;
HOSPITAL STAFF
f personnel *m* hospitalier
e personal *m* hospitalario
i personale *m* ospedaliero
n ziekenhuispersoneel *n*
d Krankenhauspersonal *n*

903 HOSPITAL MARKET
f marché *m* hospitalier
e mercado *m* hospitalario
i mercato *m* ospedaliero
n ziekenhuismarkt
d Krankenhausmarkt *m*

904 HOSPITAL MEDICAL CARE
f soins *mpl* hospitaliers médicaux
e cuidado *m* hospitalario médico
i cure *fpl* ospedaliere mediche
n medische ziekenhuisverzorging
d ärztliche Krankenhauspflege *f*;
medizinische Krankenhauspflege *f*

905 HOSPITAL MEDICAL EDUCATION
f formation *f* médicale à l'hôpital
e educación *f* médica en el hospital
i formazione *f* medica nell'ospedale
n medisch onderwijs *n* in het ziekenhuis
d medizinische Ausbildung *f* im Krankenhaus

906 HOSPITAL MEDICAL MANPOWER;
HOSPITAL MEDICAL PERSONNEL;
HOSPITAL MEDICAL STAFF
f personnel *m* médical hospitalier
e personal *m* médico hospitalario
i personale *m* medico ospedaliero
n medisch ziekenhuispersoneel *n*
d medizinisches Krankenhauspersonal *n*

907 HOSPITAL MEDICAL PERSONNEL
see: HOSPITAL MEDICAL MANPOWER

908 HOSPITAL MEDICAL STAFF
see: HOSPITAL MEDICAL MANPOWER

909 HOSPITAL MEDICINE
f médecine *f* hospitalière
e medicina *f* hospitalaria
i medicina *f* ospedaliera
n ziekenhuisgeneeskunde
d Krankenhausmedizin *f*

910 HOSPITAL MIDWIFE
f accoucheuse *f* hospitalière; sage-femme *f* hospitalière
e partera *f* (comadre *f*, comadrona *f*, matrona *f*) hospitalaria
i levatrice *f* ospedaliera
n ziekenhuisvroedvrouw; ziekenhuisverloskundige
d Krankenhaushebamme *f*; Krankenhausgeburtshelferin *f*

911 HOSPITAL MORTALITY
see: HOSPITAL DEATH RATE

912 HOSPITAL NIGHT CARE
f soins *mpl* hospitaliers de nuit
e cuidado *m* hospitalario nocturno
i cure *fpl* ospedaliere notturne
n ziekenhuis-nachtverzorging
d Krankenhausnachtversorgung *f*

913 HOSPITAL NURSE
f infirmière *f* hospitalière
e enfermera *f* hospitalaria
i infermiera *f* ospedaliera
n ziekenhuisverpleegster; ziekenhuisverpleegkundige; ziekenhuisverplegende
d Krankenhauspflegerin *f*

914 HOSPITAL NURSES' SCHOOL; HOSPITAL NURSES' TRAINING SCHOOL; HOSPITAL NURSING SCHOOL; HOSPITAL SCHOOL OF NURSING
f école *f* infirmière d'un hôpital; école *f* d'infirmières d'un hôpital; école *f* d'enseignement infirmier d'un hôpital
e escuela *f* de enfermería de un hospital; escuela *f* de (para) enfermeras de un hospital; escuela *f* de enseñanza para enfermeras de un hospital
i scuola *f* di formazione professionale per infermiere d'un ospedale
n verpleegstersschool van een ziekenhuis
d Krankenpflegeschule *f* eines Krankenhauses; Pflegerinnenschule *f* eines Krankenhauses; Schwesternschule *f* eines Krankenhauses; Schule *f* für Schwesternausbildung eines Krankenhauses

915 HOSPITAL NURSES' TRAINING SCHOOL
see: HOSPITAL NURSES' SCHOOL

916 HOSPITAL NURSING SCHOOL
see: HOSPITAL NURSES' SCHOOL

917 HOSPITAL OCCUPANCY; HOSPITAL OCCUPATION
f occupation *f* hospitalière
e ocupación *f* hospitalaria
i occupazione *f* ospedaliera
n ziekenhuisbezetting
d Krankenhausbelegung *f*

918 HOSPITAL OCCUPANCY PERCENT(AGE); HOSPITAL OCCUPANCY RATE; HOSPITAL OCCUPANCY RATIO; HOSPITAL OCCUPATION PERCENT(AGE); HOSPITAL OCCUPATION RATE; HOSPITAL OCCUPATION RATIO
f pourcentage *m* d'occupation hospitalière; taux *m* d'occupation hospitalière
e porcentaje *m* de ocupación hospitalaria; tasa *f* de ocupación hospitalaria
i percentuale *f* d'occupazione ospedaliera; tasso *m* d'occupazione ospedaliera
n ziekenhuisbezettingspercentage *n*; ziekenhuisbezettingsgraad
d prozentuale Krankenhausbelegung *f*; Krankenhausbelegungsprozentsatz *m*; Krankenhausbelegungsgrad *m*

919 HOSPITAL OCCUPANCY RATE
see: HOSPITAL OCCUPANCY PERCENT

920 HOSPITAL OCCUPANCY RATIO
see: HOSPITAL OCCUPANCY PERCENT

921 HOSPITAL OCCUPATION
see: HOSPITAL OCCUPANCY

922 HOSPITAL OCCUPATION PERCENT(AGE)
see: HOSPITAL OCCUPANCY PERCENT

923 HOSPITAL OCCUPATION RATE
see: HOSPITAL OCCUPANCY PERCENT

924 HOSPITAL OCCUPATION RATIO
see: HOSPITAL OCCUPANCY PERCENT

925 HOSPITALOGY; HOSPITAL SCIENCE
f science *f* hospitalière
e ciencia *f* hospitalaria
i scienza *f* ospedaliera
n ziekenhuiskunde; ziekenhuiswetenschap
d Krankenhauswissenschaft *f*

926 HOSPITAL ORGANIZATION
f organisation *f* hospitalière
e organización *f* hospitalaria
i organizzazione *f* ospedaliera
n ziekenhuisorganisatie
d Krankenhausorganisation *f*

927 HOSPITAL OUTPATIENT
see: AMBULATORY PATIENT

928 HOSPITAL PATIENT
f malade *m* (patient *m*) recevant des soins hospitaliers
e paciente *m* (enfermo *m*) atendido en el hospital
i malato *m* che riceve cure ospedaliere
n ziekenhuispatiënt
d Krankenhauspatient *m*

929 HOSPITAL PERIODICAL
see: HOSPITAL JOURNAL

930 HOSPITAL PERSONNEL
see: HOSPITAL MANPOWER

931 HOSPITAL PHARMACIST
f pharmacien *m* hospitalier
e farmacéutico *m* hospitalario; boticario *m* hospitalario
i farmacista *m* ospedaliero
n ziekenhuisapotheker
d Krankenhausapotheker *m*

932 HOSPITAL PHARMACY
f pharmacie *f* hospitalière
e farmacia *f* hospitalaria; botica *f* hospitalaria
i farmacia *f* ospedaliera
n ziekenhuisapotheek
d Krankenhausapotheke *f*

933 HOSPITAL PHYSICIAN
see: HOSPITAL DOCTOR

934 HOSPITAL PLAN
f plan *m* hospitalier
e plan *m* hospitalario
i piano *m* ospedaliero
n ziekenhuisplan *n*
d Krankenhausplan *m*

935 HOSPITAL PLANNING
f planification *f* hospitalière
e planificación *f* hospitalaria; planeamiento *m* hospitalario
i pianificazione *f* ospedaliera
n ziekenhuisplanning
d Krankenhausplanung *f*

936 HOSPITAL POLICY
f politique *f* hospitalière
e política *f* hospitalaria
i politica *f* ospedaliera
n ziekenhuispolitiek
d Krankenhauspolitik *f*

937 HOSPITAL POPULATION
f population *f* hospitalière
e población *f* hospitalaria
i popolazione *f* ospedaliera
n ziekenhuispopulatie
d Krankenhausbevölkerung *f*

938 HOSPITAL PRACTICE
f pratique *f* hospitalière
e práctica *f* hospitalaria
i pratica *f* ospedaliera
n ziekenhuispraktijk
d Krankenhauspraxis *f*

939 HOSPITAL PRESCRIPTION
f ordonnance *f* hospitalière
e receta *f* hospitalaria; prescripción *f* hospitalaria
i ricetta *f* ospedaliera
n ziekenhuisrecept *n*
d Krankenhausvorschrift *f*

940 HOSPITAL PROFESSION
f profession *f* hospitalière
e profesión *f* hospitalaria
i professione *f* ospedaliera
n ziekenhuisberoep *n*
d Krankenhausberuf *m*

941 HOSPITAL RECORDS
see: HOSPITAL ARCHIVES

942 HOSPITAL REFORM
f réforme *f* hospitalière
e reforma *f* hospitalaria
i riforma *f* ospedaliera
n ziekenhuishervorming
d Krankenhausreform *f*

943 HOSPITAL REGION
f région *f* hospitalière
e región *f* hospitalaria
i regione *f* ospedaliera
n ziekenhuisrayon *n*
d Krankenhauseinzugsgebiet *n*; Krankenhausversorgungsgebiet *n*

944 HOSPITAL RESEARCH
f recherche *f* hospitalière
e investigación *f* hospitalaria
i ricerca *f* ospedaliera
n ziekenhuisonderzoek *n*
d Krankenhausforschung *f*

945 HOSPITAL RESPOSIBILITY
see: HOSPITAL LIABILITY

946 HOSPITAL SCHOOL OF NURSING
see: HOSPITAL NURSES' SCHOOL

947 HOSPITAL SCIENCE
see: HOSPITALOGY

948 HOSPITAL SERVICES
see: HOSPITAL FACILITIES

949 HOSPITAL SHIP
f bateau *m* hospitalier; navire-hôpital *m*
e barco-hospital *m*
i nave-ospedale *f*
n hospitaalschip *n*
d Krankenhausschiff *n*

950 HOSPITAL SHOP
f boutique *f* hospitalière
e tienda *f* hospitalaria
i bazar *m* ospedaliero
n ziekenhuiswinkel; ziekenhuistoko
d Krankenhausladen *m*

951 HOSPITAL SIZE
f taille *f* de l'hôpital
e tamaño *m* del hospital
i capacità *f* ospedaliera
n ziekenhuisgrootte; ziekenhuisomvang
d Krankenhausgrösse *f*

952 HOSPITAL SOCIAL AID; HOSPITAL SOCIAL ASSISTANCE; HOSPITAL SOCIAL WORK
f assistance *f* sociale hospitalière; aide *f* sociale hospitalière; travail *m* social hospitalier
e asistencia *f* social hospitalaria; ayuda *f* social hospitalaria; trabajo *m* social hospitalario
i assistenza *f* sociale ospedaliera; lavoro *m* sociale ospedaliero
n maatschappelijk werk *n* in het ziekenhuis
d Krankenhaussozialhilfe *f*; Krankenhaussozialarbeit *f*; Krankenhaussozialbetreuung *f*

953 HOSPITAL SOCIAL ASSISTANCE
see: HOSPITAL SOCIAL AID

954 HOSPITAL SOCIAL SERVICE DEPARTMENT
f service *m* (département *m*) social hospitalier
e servicio *m* (departamento *m*) social hospitalario
i servizio *m* sociale ospedaliero
n sociale dienst in het ziekenhuis
d sozialer Dienst *m* im Krankenhaus; Sozialdienst *m* im Krankenhaus

955 HOSPITAL SOCIAL WORK
see: HOSPITAL SOCIAL AID

956 HOSPITAL SOCIAL WORKER
f assistant *m* social hospitalier;
travailleur *m* social hospitalier
e asistente *m* social hospitalario;
trabajador *m* social hospitalario
i assistente *m* sociale ospedaliero;
operatore *m* sociale ospedaliero
n maatschappelijk werker in het ziekenhuis;
sociaal werker in het ziekenhuis
d Krankenhaussozialfürsorger *m*;
Krankenhaussozialarbeiter *m*

957 HOSPITAL SPIRITUAL CARE
f charge *f* des âmes dans l'hôpital
e cura *f* de almas en el hospital
i cura *f* d'anime nell' ospedale
n ziekenhuiszielzorg
d Krankenhausseelsorge *f*

958 HOSPITAL STAFF
see: HOSPITAL MANPOWER

959 HOSPITAL STATISTICS
f statistique *f* hospitalière
e estadística *f* hospitalaria
i statistica *f* ospedaliera
n ziekenhuisstatistiek
d Krankenhausstatistik *f*

960 HOSPITAL STAY
f séjour *m* hospitalier
e estancia *f* hospitalaria;
estadía *f* hospitalaria
i soggiorno *m* ospedaliero
n ziekenhuisverblijf *n*
d Krankenhausaufenthalt *m*

961 HOSPITAL STRUCTURE
f structure *f* hospitalière
e estructura *f* hospitalaria
i struttura *f* ospedaliera
n ziekenhuisstructuur
d Krankenhausstruktur *f*

962 HOSPITAL SUPPLIES
f matériel *m* hospitalier;
articles *mpl* hospitaliers
e necesidades *fpl* hospitalarias;
abastecimientos *mpl* hospitalarios;
artículos *mpl* hospitalarios
i materiale *m* ospedaliero;
articoli *mpl* ospedalieri
n ziekenhuisbenodigdheden;
ziekenhuisartikelen
d Krankenhausbedarf *m*;
Krankenhausartikel *mpl*

963 HOSPITAL SYSTEM
f système *m* hospitalier
e sistema *m* hospitalario
i sistema *m* ospedaliero
n systeem *n* van ziekenhuisvoorzieningen
d Krankenhaussystem *n*

964 HOSPITAL TARIFF
see: HOSPITAL FEE

965 HOSPITAL TARIFF SETTING
see: HOSPITAL FEE SETTING

966 HOSPITAL TECHNOLOGY
f technologie *f* hospitalière
e tecnología *f* hospitalaria
i tecnologia *f* ospedaliera
n ziekenhuistechnologie
d Krankenhaustechnologie *f*

967 HOSPITAL TEXTILE
f textile *m* hospitalier
e tejido *m* hospitalario
i abbigliamento *m* ospedaliero
n ziekenhuistextiel *n*
d Krankenhaustextilien *pl*

968 HOSPITAL TRAIN
f train-hôpital *m*
e tren-hospital *m*
i treno-ospedale *m*
n ziekentrein
d Krankenzug *m*;
Sanitätszug *m*

969 HOSPITAL TREATMENT
f traitement *m* hospitalier
e tratamiento *m* hospitalario
i trattamento *m* ospedaliero
n ziekenhuisbehandeling
d Krankenhausbehandlung *f*

970 HOSPITAL TYPE
f type *m* d'hôpital
e tipo *m* de hospital
i tipo *m* d'ospedale
n ziekenhuistype *n*
d Krankenhaustyp *m*

971 HOSPITAL UNIT
f unité *f* hospitalière
e unidad *f* hospitalaria
i unità *f* ospedaliera
n ziekenhuiseenheid
d Krankenhausstation *f*

972 HOSPITAL UTILIZATION
f utilisation *f* hospitalière
e utilización *f* hospitalaria
i utilizzazione *f* ospedaliera
n ziekenhuisgebruik *n*
d Krankenhausausnutzung *f*

973 HOSPITAL WARD;
SICK WARD
f salle *f* hospitalière;
salle *f* d'hôpital;
infirmerie *f*
e sala *f* hospitalaria;
sala *f* de hospital;
crujía *f*
i sala *f* ospedaliera;
infermeria *f*
n zieken(huis)zaal
d Kranken(haus)saal *m*;
Pflegesaal *m*

974 HOSPITAL WASTE
f déchets *mpl* hospitaliers
e desechos *mpl* hospitalarios
i rifiuti *mpl* ospedalieri
n ziekenhuisafval *n*
d Krankenhausabfall *m*

975 HOT-WATER BOTTLE
f bouillotte *f*
e botella *f* caliente

i borsa *f* d'acqua calda
n bedkruik
d Wärmflasche *f*

976 HUMAN EXPERIMENTATION
f expérimentation *f* humaine
e experimentación *f* humana
i esperimento *m* umano
n menselijk experiment *n*
d Menschenversuch *m*

977 HUMAN STERILIZATION
f stérilisation *f* humaine
e esterilización *f* humana
i sterilizzazione *f* umana
n sterilisatie van mensen
d menschliche Sterilisation *f*

978 HYDROTHERAPY
f hydrothérapie *f*
e hidroterapia *f*
i idroterapia *f*
n hydrotherapie
d Hydrotherapie *f*

979 HYDROTHERAPY APPARATUS
f appareils *mpl* d'hydrothérapie
e aparatos *mpl* de hidroterapia
i apparecchi *mpl* per idroterapia
n hydrotherapie-apparatuur
d Hydrotherapiegeräte *npl*

980 HYDROTHERAPY DEPARTMENT
f service *m* (département *m*) d'hydrothérapie
e servicio *m* (departamento *m*) de hidroterapia
i servizio *m* d'idroterapia
n hydrotherapie-afdeling
d hydrotherapeutische Abteilung *f*

981 HYGIENE
f hygiène *f*
e higiene *f*
i igiene *f*
n hygiëne
d Hygiene *f*

982 HYGIENIC GYMNASTICS
f gymnastique *f* médicale
e gimnasia *f* médica
i ginnastica *f* medica
n heilgymnastiek
d Heilgymnastik *f*

983 HYPERBARIC OXYGENTHERAPY
f oxygénothérapie *f* hyperbare
e oxigenoterapia *f* hipérbara
i ossigenoterapia *f* iperbarica
n hyperbare zuurstoftherapie
d hyperbare Sauerstofftherapie *f*; Überdruck-Sauerstofftherapie *f*

984 HYPERBARIC ROOM
f chambre *f* hyperbare
e cámara *f* hipérbara
i camera *f* iperbarica
n hyperbare kamer
d Hyperbarzimmer *n*; Überdruckzimmer *n*

985 HYPERBARIC UNIT
f unité *f* hyperbare
e unidad *f* hipérbara
i unità *f* iperbarica
n hyperbare eenheid
d Hyperbarstation *f*; Überdruckstation *f*

986 HYPODERMIC NEEDLE
f aiguille *f* pour injections
e aguja *f* para poner inyecciones
i ago *m* per iniezioni
n injectienaald
d Injektionsnadel *f*

987 HYPODERMIC SYRING
f seringue *f* pour injections
e jeringa *f* para poner inyecciones
i siringa *f* per iniezioni
n injectiespuit
d Injektionsspritze *f*

I

988 ILLNESS
see: DISEASE

989 ILLNESS CLASSIFICATION
see: DISEASE CLASSIFICATION

990 ILLNESS PREVENTION
see: DISEASE PREVENTION

991 ILLNESS TRANSMISSION
see: DISEASE TRANSMISSION

992 IMMUNOLOGIST
f immunologue *m*
e inmunólogo *m*
i immunologo *m*
n immunoloog
d Immunologe *m*

993 IMMUNOLOGY
f immunologie *f*
e inmunología *f*
i immunologia *f*
n immunologie
d Immunologie *f*

994 INCUBATION ROOM
see: CULTURE ROOM

995 INCUBATOR
f couveuse *f*
e incubadora *f*
i incubatrice *f*
n couveuse
d Brutapparat *m* für Neugeborene;
Couveuse *f*

996 INDIGENT CARE
f assistance *f*
e asistencia *f* pública
i assistenza *f*
n armenzorg
d Armenpflege *f*

997 INDUSTRIAL DISEASE;
OCCUPATIONAL DISEASE
f maladie *f* professionnelle
e enfermedad *f* profesional
i malattia *f* professionale
n beroepsziekte
d Berufskrankheit *f*

998 INDUSTRIAL HEALTH SERVICE;
INDUSTRIAL MEDICAL SERVICE;
OCCUPATIONAL HEALTH SERVICE;
OCCUPATIONAL MEDICAL SERVICE
f service *m* de médecine du travail
e servicio *m* de medicina del trabajo
i servizio *m* di medicina del lavoro
n bedrijfsgeneeskundige dienst
d arbeitsmedizinischer Dienst *m*;
gewerbeärztlicher Dienst *m*

999 INDUSTRIAL HYGIENE;
OCCUPATIONAL HYGIENE
f hygiène *f* du travail
e higiene *f* del trabajo
i igiene *f* del lavoro
n arbeidshygiëne;
bedrijfshygiëne
d Arbeitshygiene *f*;
Gewerbehygiene *f*

1000 INDUSTRIAL MEDICAL SERVICE
see: INDUSTRIAL HEALTH SERVICE

1001 INDUSTRIAL MEDICINE;
OCCUPATIONAL MEDICINE
f médecine *f* du travail
e medicina *f* del trabajo
i medicina *f* dellavoro
n arbeidsgeneeskunde;
bedrijfsgeneeskunde
d Arbeitsmedizin *f*;
Gewerbemedizin *f*

1002 INDUSTRIAL NURSING;
OCCUPATIONAL NURSING
f soins *mpl* infirmiers en hygiène professionnel
e enfermería *f* de higiene profesional
i cure *fpl* infermieristiche nell'igiene professionale;
assistenza *f* infermieristica nell'igiene professionale
n bedrijfsverpleging;
bedrijfsverpleegkunde
d Betriebskrankenpflege *f*

1003 INDUSTRIAL PHYSICIAN
see: FACTORY PHYSICIAN

1004 INFANT CARE
f soins *mpl* des nourissons
e cuidado *m* (atención *f*) de los nenes
i assistenza *f* dei neonati
n zuigelingenzorg
d Säuglingspflege *f*;
Säuglingsfürsorge *f*

1005 INFANT CARE INCUBATOR
f couveuse *f* pour prématurés
e incubadora *f* para prematuros
i incubatrice *f* per neonati prematuri
n infant care couveuse
d Brutapparat *m* zur Aufzucht von Frühgeburten

1006 INFANT HEALTH CARE
f soins *mpl* sanitaires des nourissons
e cuidado *m* sanitario de los nenes
i assistenza *f* sanitaria dei neonati
n gezondheidszorg voor zuigelingen
d Gesundheitsfürsorge *f* für Säuglinge

1007 INFANT NURSE
f puéricultrice *f*
e puericultora *f*
i puericultrice *f*
n babyverzorgster
d Säuglingsschwester *f*;
Säuglingspflegerin *f*

1008 INFANTS' DEPARTMENT
f service *m* (département *m*) de nourissons
e servicio *m* (departamento *m*) para nenes
i servizio *m* per l'assistenza neonatale;
servizio *m* per l'assistenza dei neonati

n zuigelingenafdeling
d Säuglingsabteilung *f*

1009 INFANTS' HOME
f pouponnat *m*;
pouponnière *f*
e casa-cuna *f*
i asilo *m* infantile
n zuigelingentehuis *n*
d Säuglingsheim *n*;
Säuglingsbewahranstalt *f*

1010 INFANT WELFARE CENTRE (CENTER)
f bureau *m* de consultation de nourissons
e oficina *f* de consultas para nenes;
preventorio *m* para nenes
i consultorio *m* per lattanti
n consultatiebureau *n* voor zuigelingen
d Säuglingsberatungsstelle *f*

1011 INFECTION CONTROL
f lutte *f* contre les infections
e lucha *f* contra las infecciones
i lotta *f* contro le infezioni
n infectiebestrijding
d Infektionsbekämpfung *f*

1012 INFECTION PREVENTION
f prévention *f* des infections
e prevención *f* de infecciones
i prevenzione *f* delle infezioni
n voorkoming van infecties
d Infektionsverhütung *f*

1013 INFECTIOUS DISEASE
see: COMMUNICABLE DISEASE

1014 INFECTIOUS DISEASE CARE
see: COMMUNICABLE DISEASE CARE

1015 INFECTIOUS DISEASE CLINIC
see: COMMUNICABLE DISEASE CLINIC

1016 INFECTIOUS DISEASE CONTROL
see: COMMUNICABLE DISEASE CONTROL

1017 INFECTIOUS DISEASE DEPARTMENT
see: COMMUNICABLE DISEASE DEPARTMENT

1018 INFECTIOUS DISEASE HOSPITAL
see: COMMUNICABLE DISEASE HOSPITAL

1019 INFECTIOUS DISEASE NURSING
see: COMMUNICABLE DISEASE NURSING

1020 INFECTIOUS DISEASE UNIT
see: COMMUNICABLE DISEASE UNIT

1021 INFECTIOUS PATIENT
see: COMMUNICABLE PATIENT

1022 INHALATION THERAP(EUT)IST;
RESPIRATORY THERAP(EUT)IST
f thérapeute *m* respiratoire
e terapeuta *m* respiratorio
i fisioterapista *m* dell' apparato respiratorio
n ademhalingstherapeut
d Atemtherapeut *m*

1023 INHALATION THERAPY;
RESPIRATORY THERAPY
f thérapie *f* respiratoire
e terapia *f* respiratoria
i terapia *f* respiratoria
n ademhalingstherapie
d Atemtherapie *f*

1024 INHALATION THERAPY DEPARTMENT;
RESPIRATORY THERAPY DEPARTMENT
f service *m* (département *m*) de thérapie respiratoire
e servicio *m* (departamento *m*) de terapia respiratoria
i servizio *m* di terapia respiratoria
n ademhalingstherapie-afdeling
d Atemtherapie-Abteilung *f*

1025 INPATIENT
see: BED PATIENT

1026 INPATIENT ADMISSION
see: ADMISSION

1027 INPATIENT BED
f lit *m* d'hospitalisation
e cama *f* para pacientes (enfermos) internados
i letto *m* d'ospedalizzazione
n klinisch bed *n*
d Bett *n* für stationäre Patienten (Kranke)

1028 INPATIENT CARE
see: CLINICAL CARE

1029 INPATIENT CARE UNIT;
INPATIENT UNIT;
NURSING UNIT;
PATIENT CARE UNIT;
PATIENT UNIT
f unité *f* de soins
e unidad *f* de enfermería
i unità *f* di cure
n verpleegeenheid
d Pflegestation *f*;
Krankenstation *f*;
Bettenstation *f*;
Pflegeeinheit *f*

1030 INPATIENT CENSUS
f nombre *m* des rationnaires
e número *m* de pacientes (enfermos)
i numero *m* delle razioni
n aantal *n* opgenomen patiënten
d Zahl *f* der zu verpflegenden Patienten

1031 INPATIENT DAY
see: DAY OF CARE

1032 INPATIENT DISCHARGE
see: DISCHARGE

1033 INPATIENT FACILITIES
f services *mpl* d'hospitalisation
e servicios *mpl* para pacientes (enfermos) internados
i servizi *mpl* d'ospedalizzazione
n voorzieningen voor klinische gezondheidszorg
d stationäres Gesundheitswesen *n*

1034 INPATIENT HEALTH CARE
see: CLINICAL HEALTH CARE

1035 INPATIENT HOSPITALIZATION
see: HOSPITALIZATION

1036 INPATIENT SERVICE DAY
see: DAY OF CARE

1037 INPATIENT TREATMENT
see: CLINICAL TREATMENT

1038 INPATIENT UNIT
see: INPATIENT CARE UNIT

1039 INSECT CONTROL;
VERMIN CONTROL
f lutte *f* contre les insectes
e lucha *f* contra los insectos
i lotta *f* contro gli insetti
n insectenbestrijding;
ongediertebestrijding
d Schädlingsbekämpfung *f*;
Insektenschutz *m*

1040 INSTITUTIONAL CARE;
INTRAMURAL CARE
f soins m*pl* intra-hospitaliers;
soins *mpl* intra-muros
e cuidado *m* intra-hospitalario;
atención *f* (asistencia *f*) intra-hospitalaria;
cuidado *m* (atención *f*, asistencia *f*) institucional
i cure *fpl* intra-ospedaliere;
assistenza *f* intra-ospedaliera
n intramurale zorg;
institutionele zorg;
residentiële zorg
d Anstaltspflege *f*;
Anstaltsbetreuung *f*;
intramurale Pflege *f*

1041 INSTITUTIONAL HEALTH CARE;
INTRAMURAL HEALTH CARE
f soins *mpl* sanitaires intra-hospitaliers;
soins *mpl* sanitaires intra-muros
e cuidado *m* sanitario intra-hospitalario;
atención *f* (asistencia *f*) sanitaria intra-hospitalaria;
cuidado *m* sanitario institucional;
atención *f* (asistencia *f*) sanitaria institucional
i cure *fpl* sanitarie intra-ospedaliere;
assistenza *f* sanitaria intra-ospedaliera
n intramurale gezondheidszorg;
institutionele gezondheidszorg
d Anstaltsgesundheitsfürsorge *f*

1042 INSTITUTIONAL HEALTH CARE SERVICES;
INSTITUTIONAL HEALTH SERVICES;
INTRAMURAL HEALTH CARE SERVICES;
INTRAMURAL HEALTH SERVICES
f services *mpl* de soins intra-hospitaliers;
services *mpl* sanitaires intra-hospitaliers
e servicios *mpl* sanitarios intra-hospitalarios;
servicios *mpl* sanitarios institucionales
i servizi *mpl* sanitari ospedalieri
n diensten voor intramurale gezondheidszorg
d Anstaltspflegedienste *mpl*

1043 INSTITUTIONAL HEALTH SERVICES
see: INSTITUTIONAL HEALTH CARE SERVICES

1044 INSTITUTIONALIZATION
see: HOSPITALIZATION

1045 INSTITUTION FOR MENTALLY DEFECTIVE
see: HOSPITAL FOR MENTALLY DEFECTIVE

1046 INSTITUTION FOR MENTALLY DEFICIENT
see: HOSPITAL FOR MENTALLY DEFECTIVE

1047 INSTITUTION FOR MENTALLY HANDICAPPED
see: HOSPITAL FOR MENTALLY DEFECTIVE

1048 INSTITUTION FOR MENTALLY RETARDED
see: HOSPITAL FOR MENTALLY DEFECTIVE

1049 INSTITUTION FOR MENTALLY SUBNORMAL
see: HOSPITAL FOR MENTALLY DEFECTIVE

1050 INSURANCE MEDICINE
f médecine *f* d'assurance
e medicina *f* de seguro
i medicina *f* delle assicurazioni
n verzekeringsgeneeskunde
d Versicherungsmedizin *f*

1051 INSURANCE PHYSICIAN
f médecin *m* d'assurance
e médico *m* de seguros
i medico *m* d'assicurazione
n verzekeringsgeneeskundige
d Versicherungsarzt *m*

1052 INTENSIVE CARE
see: HIGH CARE

1053 INTENSIVE CARE APPARATUS
f appareils *mpl* de contrôle intense
e aparatos *mpl* de cuidado intensivo
i apparecchi *mpl* di controllo intensivo
n apparatuur voor intensieve bewaking
d Intensivüberwachungsgeräte *npl*

1054 INTENSIVE CARE DEPARTMENT
see: HIGH CARE DEPARTMENT

1055 INTENSIVE CARE INCUBATOR
f couveuse *f* de contrôle intensif
e incubadora *f* de cuidado intensivo
i incubatrice *f* per il controllo intensivo
n intensive care couveuse
d Intensivüberwachungsbrutapparat *m*

1056 INTENSIVE CARE NURSE
f infirmière *f* de soins intensifs
e enfermera *f* de cuidado intensivo
i infermiera *f* per cure intensive
n intensive care verpleegkundige
d Intensivpflegeschwester *f*

1057 INTENSIVE CARE UNIT
see: HIGH CARE UNIT

1058 INTENSIVE MEDICINE
f médecine *f* intensive
e medicina *f* intensiva
i medicina *f* intensiva
n intensieve geneeskunde
d Intensivmedizin *f*

1059 INTENSIVE PSYCHIATRIC CARE
f soins *mpl* psychiatriques intensifs
e cuidado *m* psiquiátrico intensivo
i cure *fpl* psichiatriche intensive
n intensieve psychiatrische zorg
d intensive psychiatrische Versorgung *f*

1060 INTENSIVE TREATMENT
f traitement *m* intensif
e tratamiento *m* intensivo
i trattamento *m* intensivo
n intensieve behandeling
d Intensivbehandlung *f*

1061 INTERFERENCE THERAPY
f thérapie *f* d'interférence
e terapia *f* de interferencia
i terapia *f* d'interferenza
n interferentietherapie
d Interferenztherapie *f*

1062 INTERMEDIATE CARE;
MEDIUM CARE;
MIDDLE CARE;
NORMAL CARE
f soins *mpl* courants
e cuidado *m* (atención *f*) corriente;
cuidado *m* (atención *f*) intermedio(a);
cuidado *m* (atención *f*) normal
i cure *fpl* correnti;
cure *fpl* normali
n middenzorg
d Normalpflege *f*

1063 INTERMEDIATE CARE DEPARTMENT
f service *m* (département *m*) de soins courants
e servicio *m* (departamento *m*) de cuidado corriente
i servizio *m* di cure correnti
n afdeling voor middenzorg
d Normalpflegeabteilung *f*

1064 INTERMITTENT CARE
f soins *mpl* intermittents
e cuidado *m* (atención *f*) intermitente
i cure *fpl* intermittenti
n intermitterende zorg
d intermittierende Pflege *f*

1065 INTERNAL MEDICINE
f médecine *f* interne
e medicina *f* interna
i medicina *f* interna
n interne geneeskunde;
inwendige geneeskunde
d innere Medizin *f*

1066 INTERNIST;
MEDICAL DOCTOR
f médecin *m* interniste;
médecin *m* de médecine interne;
spécialiste *m* pour les maladies internes
e médico *m* para enfermedades internas
i medico *m* internista;
specialista *m* in medicina interna
n internist
d Internist *m*;
Arzt *m* für innere Krankheiten

1067 INTRAMURAL CARE
see: INSTITUTIONAL CARE

1068 INTRAMURAL HEALTH CARE
see: INSTITUTIONAL HEALTH CARE

1069 INTRAMURAL HEALTH CARE SERVICES
see: INSTITUTIONAL HEALTH CARE SERVICES

1070 INTRAMURAL HEALTH SERVICES
see: INSTITUTIONAL HEALTH CARE SERVICES

1071 INTRAVENOUS THERAPY
f thérapie *f* intraveineuse
e terapia *f* intravenosa
i terapia *f* endovenosa
n intraveneuse therapie
d intravenöse Therapie *f*

1072 INVALID CARRIAGE
f voiture *f* d'invalide
e coche *m* de inválidos
i vettura *f* per invalidi
n invalidenwagen
d Invalidenwagen *m*;
Krankenfahrstuhl *m*

1073 INVALIDITY INSURANCE
see: DISABLEMENT INSURANCE

1074 IODINE ROOM
f salle *f* d'iode
e sala *f* de yodo
i sala *f* per l'impiego dello iodio
n jodiumkamer
d Jodraum *m*

1075 ISOLATING BOX
f box *m* d'isolement
e box *m* de aislamiento
i padiglione *m* d'isolamento
n isoleerbox
d Isolierbox *m*

1076 ISOLATION DEPARTMENT
f service *m* (département *m*) d'isolement
e servicio *m* (departamento *m*) de aislamiento
i divisione *f* d'isolamento
n isoleerafdeling
d Isolierabteilung *f*

1077 ISOLATION HOSPITAL
f hôpital *m* d'isolement
e hospital *m* de aislamiento
i ospedale *m* d'isolamento
n isoleerziekenhuis *n*
d Isolierkrankenhaus *n*

1078 ISOLATION ROOM
f chambre *f* d'isolement
e habitación *f* de aislamiento
i camera *f* d'isolamento
n isoleerkamer
d Isolierzimmer *n*

1079 ISOLATION UNIT
f unité *f* d'isolement
e unidad *f* de aislamiento
i unità *f* d'isolamento
n isoleereenheid
d Isolierstation *f*

1080 ISOTOPE LABORATORY
f laboratoire *m* d'isotopes
e laboratorio *m* de isotopos
i laboratorio *m* di isotopi
n isotopenlaboratorium *n*
d Isotopenlaboratorium *n*

J

1081 JAW SURGERY;
MAXILLARY SURGERY
f chirurgie *f* maxillaire
e cirugía *f* maxilar
i chirurgia *f* maxillo-facciale
n kaakchirurgie
d Kieferchirurgie *f*

K

1082 KIDNEY BANK
f banque *f* de reins
e banco *m* de riñones
i banca *f* dei reni
n nierbank
d Nierenbank *f*

1083 KINESITHERAP(EUT)IST
f kinésithérapeute *m*
e cinesiterapeuta *m*
i chinesi(o)terapista *m*
n kinesitherapeut; bewegingstherapeut
d Kinesitherapeut *m*; Bewegungstherapeut *m*

1084 KINESITHERAPY
f kinésithérapie *f*
e cinesiterapia *f*
i chinesi(o)terapia *f*
n kinesitherapie; bewegingstherapie
d Kinesitherapie *f*; Bewegungstherapie *f*

1085 KITCHENETTE
f cuisinette *f*
e cocinita *f*
i cucinino *m*
n theekeuken
d Teeküche *f*

L

1086 LABORATORY
f laboratoire *m*
e laboratorio *m*
i laboratorio *m*
n laboratorium *n*
d Laboratorium *n*

1087 LABORATORY APPARATUS
f appareils *mpl* de laboratoire
e aparatos *mpl* de laboratorio
i apparecchi *mpl* di laboratorio
n laboratoriumapparatuur
d Laboratoriumgeräte *npl*

1088 LABORATORY MEDICINE
f médecine *f* de laboratoire
e medicina *f* de laboratorio
i medicina *f* di laboratorio
n laboratoriumgeneeskunde
d Laboratoriummedizin *f*

1089 LABORATORY TECHNICIAN
f technicien *m* de laboratoire
e técnico *m* de laboratorio
i tecnico *m* di laboratorio
n laboratoriumtechnicus
d Laboratoriumtechniker *m*

1090 LABOUR ROOM
f chambre *f* de travail préparatoire à l'accouchement
e cuarto *m* de trabajo
i sala *f* di preparazione al parto
n voorbereidingskamer voor de bevalling
d Vorbereitungsraum *m* für die Entbindung

1091 LARGE HOSPITAL
f grand hôpital *m*
e gran hospital *m*
i grande ospedale *m*
n groot ziekenhuis *n*
d Grosskrankenhaus *n*

1092 LAVATORY BED
f lit *m* pour incontinents
e cama *f* para incontinentes
i letto *m* per incontinenti
n closetbed *n*
d Klosettbett *n*

1093 LAVATORY MATTRESS
f matelas *m* pour incontinents
e colchón *m* para incontinentes
i materasso *m* per incontinenti
n closetmatras
d Klosettmatratze *f*

1094 LENGTH OF HOSPITALIZATION
see: DURATION OF HOSPITALIZATION

1095 LENGTH OF STAY
see: DURATION OF HOSPITALIZATION

1096 LEPER HOSPITAL
f léproserie *f*
e leprosería *f*;
hospital *m* de leprosos
i lebbrosario *m*
n leprozenhuis *n*
d Leprosenhaus *n*

1097 LEVEL OF CARE
f niveau *m* des soins
e nivel *m* de cuidado (atención)
i livello *m* delle cure
n niveau *n* van de zorg
d Pflegeniveau *n*

1098 LIFE INSURANCE
f assurance *f* sur la vie
e seguro *m* sobre la vida;
seguro *m* de vida
i assicurazione *f* sulla vita
n levensverzekering
d Lebensversicherung *f*

1099 LIGHT LOCK
see: AIR LOCK

1100 LIMB BATH
f bain *m* pour membres
e baño *m* para miembros
i bagno *m* per gambe e braccia;
bagno *m* per arti
n deelbad *n*
d Teilbad *n*

1101 LINEN STORE
f entrepôt *m* de linge
e depósito *m* de ropa
i deposito *m* della biancheria;
guardaroba *m*
n schoonlinnenopslag
d Wäschelager *n*

1102 LOCAL HOSPITAL
f hôpital *m* local
e hospital *m* local
i ospedale *m* generale zonale
n lokaal ziekenhuis *n*;
plaatselijk ziekenhuis *n*
d Ortskrankenhaus *n*;
örtliches Krankenhaus *n*

1103 LOGOPEDICS;
SPEECH THERAPY
f logopédie *f*;
éducation *f* phonétique
e logopedia *f*
i rieducazione *f* fonetica
n logopedie;
spraaktherapie
d Logopädie *f*;
Sprachheilbehandlung *f*;
Sprachheilkunde *f*

1104 LOGOPEDICS DEPARTMENT;
SPEECH THERAPY DEPARTMENT
f service *m* (département *m*) de logopédie
e servicio *m* (departamento *m*) de logopedia
i servizio *m* di logopedia
n logopedie-afdeling
d Logopädieabteilung *f*

1105 LONG STAY CARE
see: CHRONIC CARE

1106 LONG STAY CARE INSTITUTION
see: CHRONIC CARE INSTITUTION

1107 LONG STAY DEPARTMENT
see: CHRONIC ILLNESS DEPARTMENT

1108 LONG STAY FACILITIES
see: CHRONIC DISEASE FACILITIES

1109 LONG STAY HOSPITAL
see: CHRONIC CARE INSTITUTION

1110 LONG STAY HOSPITAL CARE;
LONG TERM HOSPITAL CARE
f soins *mpl* hospitaliers de longue durée
e cuidado *m* hospitalario a largo plazo;
atención *f* hospitalaria a largo plazo
i cure *fpl* ospedaliere di lunga durata
n langdurige ziekenhuisverpleging
d langfristige Krankenhauspflege *f*

1111 LONG STAY INSTITUTION
see: CHRONIC CARE INSTITUTION

1112 LONG STAY NURSING
see: CHRONIC ILLNESS NURSING

1113 LONG STAY PATIENT
see: CHRONIC PATIENT

1114 LONG STAY PATIENT CARE
see: CHRONIC CARE

1115 LONG STAY UNIT
see: CHRONIC ILLNESS UNIT

1116 LONG TERM CARE
see: CHRONIC CARE

1117 LONG TERM CARE INSTITUTION
see: CHRONIC CARE INSTITUTION

1118 LONG TERM DEPARTMENT
see: CHRONIC ILLNESS DEPARTMENT

1119 LONG TERM DISEASE
see: CHRONIC DISEASE

1120 LONG TERM FACILITIES
see: CHRONIC DISEASE FACILITIES

1121 LONG TERM HOSPITAL
see: CHRONIC CARE INSTITUTION

1122 LONG TERM HOSPITAL CARE
see: LONG STAY HOSPITAL CARE

1123 LONG TERM ILLNESS
see: CHRONIC DISEASE

1124 LONG TERM INSTITUTION
see: CHRONIC CARE INSTITUTION

1125 LONG TERM NURSING
see: CHRONIC ILLNESS NURSING

1126 LONG TERM PATIENT
see: CHRONIC PATIENT

1127 LONG TERM PATIENT CARE
see: CHRONIC CARE

1128 LONG TERM SICKNESS
see: CHRONIC DISEASE

1129 LONG TERM THERAPY
f thérapie *f* de longue durée
e terapia *f* de larga duración
i terapia *f* di lunga durata
n langdurige therapie
d Langzeittherapie *f*

1130 LONG TERM UNIT
see: CHRONIC ILLNESS UNIT

1131 LOW CARE;
MINIMAL CARE
f soins *mpl* minima
e cuidado *m* mínimo;
atención *f* mínima
i cure *fpl* di lieve intensità
n minimale zorg
d Minimalpflege *f*;
Minimumpflege *f*;
Mindestpflege *f*;
Leichtpflege *f*

1132 LOW CARE DEPARTMENT;
MINIMAL CARE DEPARTMENT
f service *m* (département *m*) de soins minima
e servicio *m* (departamento *m*) de cuidado mínimo
i servizio *m* di cure di lieve intensità
n afdeling voor minimale zorg
d Minimalpflegeabteilung *f*

1133 LOW CARE PATIENT;
MINIMAL CARE PATIENT
f malade *m* (patient *m*) de soins minima
e paciente *m* (enfermo *m*) de cuidado mínimo
i malato *m* che abbisogna di cure di lieve intensità
n patiënt met minimale verzorgingsbehoefte
d Minimalpflegepatient *m*

1134 LOW CARE UNIT;
MINIMAL CARE UNIT
f unité *f* de soins minima
e unidad *f* de cuidado mínimo
i unità *f* di cure di lieve intensità
n eenheid voor minimale zorg
d Minimalpflegestation *f*

M

1135 MALE NURSE
see: ATTENDANT

1136 MARINE THERAPY;
THALASSOTHERAPY
f thérapie *f* marine;
thalassothérapie *f*
e terapia *f* marina;
talasoterapia *f*
i talassoterapia *f*
n zeetherapie;
thalassotherapie
d Seetherapie *f*;
Thalassotherapie *f*

1137 MASSAGE ROOM
f salle *f* de massage
e sala *f* de masaje
i sala *f* per massaggi
n massageruimte
d Massageraum *m*

1138 MASS RADIOGRAPHY;
MASS X-RAY EXAMINATION
f examen *m* radiographique en série
e examen *m* radiológico de grupos
i esame *m* radiologico collettivo
n röntgenonderzoek *n* van de bevolking
d Röntgenreihenuntersuchung *f*

1139 MASS X-RAY EXAMINATION
see: MASS RADIOGRAPHY

1140 MATERNAL PROTECTION;
MATERNITY PROTECTION
f protection *f* maternelle
e protección *f* de la maternidad
i protezione *f* della maternità
n moederschapszorg
d Mutterschutz *m*

1141 MATERNITY BED
see: CHILD BED

1142 MATERNITY CARE
f soins *mpl* de la maternité;
soins *mpl* aux accouchées
e cuidado *m* (atención *f*) de la maternidad;
cuidado *m* (atención *f*) maternal;
cuidado *m* (atención *f*) de la parturiente
i cura *f* delle partorienti
n kraamzorg;
kraamverzorging
d Wöchnerinnenpflege *f*;
Wochenpflege *f*;
Wöchnerinnenfürsorge *f*

1143 MATERNITY CENTRE (CENTER)
f centre *m* maternel;
centre *m* de protection maternelle et infantile
e centro *m* de maternidad;
consultorio *m* de maternidad
i centro *m* per la protezione della maternità e dell' infanzia
n kraamcentrum *n*;
consultatiebureau *n* voor moeders en zuigelingen
d Mütterberatungsstelle *f*;
Zentrum *n* für Mütter- und Säuglingsberatung

1144 MATERNITY CLINIC;
OBSTETRIC CLINIC
f clinique *f* de maternité;
clinique *f* d'obstétrique;
clinique *f* d'accouchement
e clínica *f* de maternidad;
clínica *f* de obstetricia
i clinica *f* di ostetricia e ginecologia
n kraam(vrouwen)kliniek;
verloskundige kliniek
d Geburtshilfeklinik *f*;
Entbindungsklinik *f*

1145 MATERNITY DEPARTMENT;
OBSTETRIC DEPARTMENT
f service *m* (département *m*) de maternité;
service *m* (département *m*) d'obstétrique;
service *m* (département *m*) d'accouchement
e servicio *m* (departamento *m*) de maternidad;
servicio *m* (departamento *m*) de obstetricia
i divisione *f* di ostetricia e ginecologia
n kraam(vrouwen)afdeling;
verloskundige afdeling
d Geburtshilfeabteilung *f*;
Entbindungsabteilung *f*

1146 MATERNITY HOSPITAL;
OBSTETRIC HOSPITAL
f maternité *f*;
maison *f* d'accouchement
e casa *f* de maternidad;
maternidad *f*;
hospital *m* matriz;
hospital *m* para obstetricia
i maternità *f*
n kraaminrichting
d Entbindungsanstalt *f*;
Entbindungsheim *n*;
Gebäranstalt *f*;
Wöchnerinnenheim *n*

1147 MATERNITY MORTALITY
f mortalité *f* d'accouchées
e mortalidad *f* de parturientes
i mortalità *f* delle partorienti
n kraamvrouwensterfte
d Wöchnerinnenmortalität *f*

1148 MATERNITY NURSE;
OBSTETRIC NURSE
f garde-couches *f*;
infirmière *f* obstétricienne
e enfermera *f* obstétrica
i ostetrica *f*
n kraamverpleegster
d Wochenbettpflegerin *f*;
Wochenpflegerin *f*;
Hebammenschwester *f*

1149 MATERNITY NURSING;
OBSTETRIC NURSING
f soins *mpl* infirmiers de maternité
e enfermería *f* de maternidad
i cure *fpl* di maternità
n kraamverpleging
d Wochenbettpflege *f*

1150 MATERNITY PATIENT
f accouchée *f*
e parturiente *f*
i partoriente *f*
n kraamvrouw
d Wöchnerin *f*;
Kindbetterin *f*

1151 MATERNITY PROTECTION
see: MATERNAL PROTECTION

1152 MATERNITY SERVICES
f services *mpl* de maternité
e servicios *mpl* de maternidad
i servizi *mpl* di ostetricia e ginecologia
n kraamdiensten
d Geburtshilfedienste *mpl*

1153 MATERNITY UNIT;
OBSTETRIC UNIT
f unité *f* de maternité;
unité *f* d'obstétrique;
unité *f* d'accouchement
e unidad *f* de maternidad;
unidad *f* de obstetricia
i unità *f* di ostetricia e ginecologia
n kraam(vrouwen)eenheid;
verloskundige eenheid
d Geburtshilfestation *f*;
Entbindungsstation *f*

1154 MATRON
see: HEAD OF THE NURSING SERVICE

1155 MAXILLARY SURGERY
see: JAW SURGERY

1156 MAXIMUM CARE
see: HIGH CARE

1157 MEALS DISTRIBUTION
see: FOOD DISTRIBUTION

1158 MECHANOTHERAPY
f mécanothérapie *f*
e mecanoterapia *f*
i meccanoterapia *f*
n mechanotherapie
d Mechanotherapie *f*

1159 MEDICAL ABSENTEEISM
see: ABSENCE DUE TO SICKNESS

1160 MEDICAL ADMINISTRATION
f administration *f* médicale
e administración *f* médica
i amministrazione *f* medica
n medische administratie
d medizinische Verwaltung *f*

1161 MEDICAL ANALYSES LABORATORY
f laboratoire *m* d'analyses médicales
e laboratorio *m* de análisis médicos
i laboratorio *m* d'analisi mediche
n laboratorium *n* voor medische analyses
d Laboratorium *n* für medizinische Analysen

1162 MEDICAL APPARATUS
f appareils *mpl* médicaux
e aparatos *mpl* médicos
i apparecchi *mpl* medici
n medische apparatuur
d medizinische Geräte *npl*

1163 MEDICAL ARCHIVES;
MEDICAL FILES;
MEDICAL RECORDS
f archives *fpl* médicales
e archivo *m* médico
i archivi *mpl* medici
n medisch archief *n*
d ärztliches Archiv *n*;
medizinisches Archiv *n*

1164 MEDICAL ASSISTANCE;
MEDICAL HELP
f assistance *f* médicale;
aide *f* médicale
e ayuda *f* médica
i assistenza *f* medica
n medische hulp(verlening)
d ärztliche Hilfe *f*

1165 MEDICAL AUDIT
f contrôle *m* de la qualité des soins médicaux
e auditoria *f* médica;
evaluación *f* del cuidado médico
i controllo *m* della qualità delle cure mediche
n medical audit;
kwaliteitsmeting van de medische zorg
d Qualitätskontrolle *f* der ärztlichen Versorgung

1166 MEDICAL BATH;
MEDICINAL BATH
f bain *m* médical;
bain *m* curatif
e baño *m* medicinal
i bagno *m* terapeutico
n geneeskrachtig bad *n*
d medizinisches Bad *n*;
Heilbad *n*

1167 MEDICAL BIOLOGY
f biologie *f* médicale
e biología *f* médica
i biologia *f* medica
n medische biologie
d medizinische Biologie *f*

1168 MEDICAL BLOCK;
TREATMENT BLOCK
f bloc *m* hospitalier;
bloc *m* d'hospitalisation;
bloc *m* des services d'hospitalisation;
bâtiment *m* des lits;
bloc *m* de traitement
e bloque *m* de hospitalización;
bloque *m* de atención médica;
bloque *m* de tratamiento
i monoblocco *m*;
blocco *m* dei servizi d'ospedalizzazione;
blocco *m* di trattamento
n behandelhuis *n*;
behandelgebouw *n*;
beddenhuis *n*
d Behandlungsblock *m*;
Behandlungsbau *m*;
Betten(hoch)haus *n*

1169 MEDICAL CARE
f soins *mpl* médicaux
e cuidado *m* médico;
atención *f* (asistencia *f*) médica
i cure *fpl* mediche
n medische zorg;
medische verzorging

d ärztliche Versorgung *f*;
ärztliche Betreuung *f*;
medizinische Versorgung *f*;
medizinische Betreuung *f*

1170 MEDICAL CARE CONSUMPTION;
MEDICAL CONSUMPTION
f consommation *f* de soins médicaux;
consommation *f* médicale
e consumo *m* de cuidado médico
i l'usufruire *m* di cure mediche
n consumptie van medische zorg
d Konsum *m* ärztlicher Versorgung

1171 MEDICAL CASENOTES;
MEDICAL DATA
f données *fpl* médicales
e historias *fpl* médicas
i dati *mpl* medici
n medische gegevens
d Krankengeschichten *fpl*;
Krankenakten *fpl*

1172 MEDICAL CENTRE (CENTER)
f centre *m* médical;
centre *m* de médecine
e centro *m* médico
i centro *m* medico
n medisch centrum *n*
d medizinisches Zentrum *n*

1173 MEDICAL CERTIFICATE
f certificat *m* médical;
attestation *f* médicale
e certificado *m* de sanidad;
certificado *m* de buena salud
i certificato *m* medico
n gezondheidsattest *n*
d Gesundheitszeugnis *n*

1174 MEDICAL CHIEF
see: CHIEF DOCTOR

1175 MEDICAL CLERK;
MEDICAL SECRETARY
f secrétaire *m* médical;
secrétaire *f* médicale
e secretario *m* médico;
secretaria *f* médica
i segretario *m* medico;
segretaria *f* medica
n medisch secretaris;
medisch secretaresse
d ärztlicher Sekretär *m*;
ärztliche Sekretärin *f*

1176 MEDICAL CLINIC
f clinique *f* médicale
e clínica *f* médica
i clinica *f* medica
n medische kliniek
d medizinische Klinik *f*

1177 MEDICAL CONFIDENTIALITY;
MEDICAL SECRET
f secret *m* médical
e secreto *m* médico
i segreto *m* medico
n medisch (beroeps)geheim *n*
d ärztliches Geheimnis *n*

1178 MEDICAL CONSULTANT;
MEDICAL CONTROLLER
f médecin *m* contrôleur
e médico *m* de confianza
i medico *m* controllore;
ispettore *m* sanitario
n controlerend geneesheer
d Vertrauensarzt *m*

1179 MEDICAL CONSUMPTION
see: MEDICAL CARE CONSUMPTION

1180 MEDICAL CONTROL;
MEDICAL SUPERVISION
f contrôle *m* médical;
surveillance *f* médicale
e control *m* médico;
supervigilancia *f* médica
i controllo *m* medico;
sorveglianza *f* medica
n medische controle;
medische bewaking
d ärztliche Überwachung *f*

1181 MEDICAL CONTROLLER
see: MEDICAL CONSULTANT

1182 MEDICAL DATA
see: MEDICAL CASENOTES

1183 MEDICAL DEPARTMENT
f service *m* (département *m*) médical;
service *m* (département *m*) de médecine
e servicio *m* (departamento *m*) de medicina;
servicio *m* (departamento *m*) médico
i servizio *m* medico;
servizio *m* di medicina
n medische afdeling
d medizinische Abteilung *f*;
ärztliche Abteilung *f*

1184 MEDICAL DIAGNOSTIC LABORATORY
f laboratoire *m* de diagnostic médical
e laboratorio *m* de diagnóstico médico
i laboratorio *m* di diagnostica medica
n medisch-diagnostisch laboratorium *n*
d medizinisch-diagnostisches Laboratorium *n*

1185 MEDICAL DIRECTOR
see: CHIEF MEDICAL OFFICER

1186 MEDICAL DISCIPLINE
f discipline *f* médicale
e disciplina *f* médica
i disciplina *f* medica
n medische discipline
d medizinische Disziplin *f*

1187 MEDICAL DISPOSABLES
f articles *mpl* médicaux à usage unique
e artículos *mpl* médicos de un solo uso
i articoli *mpl* medici da usarsi una sola volta
n medische wegwerpartikelen
d medizinische Einwegartikel *mpl*;
medizinische Einmalartikel *mpl*

1188 MEDICAL DOCTOR
see: INTERNIST

1189 MEDICAL DOCUMENTATION
f documentation *f* médicale
e documentación *f* médica

i documentazione *f* medica
n medische documentatie
d medizinische Dokumentation *f*

1190 MEDICAL DOSSIER;
MEDICAL FILE
f dossier *m* médical
e expediente *m* médico
i cartella *f* medica
n medisch dossier *n*
d ärztlicher Dossier *m*;
medizinischer Dossier *m*

1191 MEDICAL ECOLOGY
f écologie *f* médicale
e ecología *f* médica
i ecologia *f* medica
n medische ecologie
d medizinische Ekologie *f*

1192 MEDICAL ECONOMICS
f économie *f* médicale
e economía *f* médica
i economia *f* medica
n medische economie
d medizinische Wirtschaft *f*

1193 MEDICAL EDUCATION;
MEDICAL INSTRUCTION;
MEDICAL TEACHING;
MEDICAL TRAINING
f formation *f* médicale;
enseignement *m* médical;
enseignement *m* de la médecine
e educación *f* médica;
enseñanza *f* médica;
enseñanza *f* en medicina
i formazione *f* medica;
insegnamento *m* della medicina
n medische opleiding;
medisch onderwijs *n*
d ärztliche Ausbildung *f*;
medizinische Ausbildung *f*;
ärztlicher Unterricht *m*;
medizinischer Unterricht *m*

1194 MEDICAL ELECTRONICS
f électronique *f* médicale
e electrónica *f* médica
i elettronica *f* medica
n medische electronica
d medizinische Elektronik *f*

1195 MEDICAL ENGINEERING;
MEDICAL TECHNIQUE
f technique *f* médicale
e técnica *f* médica
i tecnica *f* medica
n medische techniek
d medizinische Technik *f*

1196 MEDICAL EQUIPMENT
f équipement *m* médical
e equipo *m* médico
i equipaggiamento *m* medico
n medische uitrusting
d medizinische Ausrüstung *f*

1197 MEDICAL ERROR
f faute *f* médicale
e falta *f* médica
i errore *m* medico
n medische fout
d ärztlicher Fehler *m*

1198 MEDICAL ETHICS
f éthique *f* médicale
e ética *f* médica
i etica *f* medica
n medische ethiek
d ärztliche Ethik *f*

1199 MEDICAL EXAMINATION
f examen *m* médical
e examen *m* médico;
reconocimiento *m* médico
i esame *m* medico
n medisch onderzoek *n*
d ärztliche Untersuchung *f*

1200 MEDICAL FACULTY;
MEDICAL SCHOOL
f faculté *f* médicale;
faculté *f* de médecine
e facultad *f* médica;
facultad *f* de medicina
i facoltà *f* di medicina
n medische faculteit
d medizinische Fakultät *f*

1201 MEDICAL FEE
see: DOCTOR'S FEE

1202 MEDICAL FILE
see: MEDICAL DOSSIER

1203 MEDICAL FILES
see: MEDICAL ARCHIVES

1204 MEDICAL GAS
f gaz *m* médical
e gas *m* medicinal
i gas *m* medicinale
n medicinaal gas *n*;
medisch gas *n*
d medizinisches Gas *n*

1205 MEDICAL HELP
see: MEDICAL ASSISTANCE

1206 MEDICAL HISTORY
see: HISTORY OF MEDICINE

1207 MEDICAL HOSPITAL KNOWLEDGE;
MEDICAL HOSPITALOGY;
MEDICAL HOSPITAL SCIENCE
f science *f* médicale hospitalière
e ciencia *f* médico-hospitalaria
i scienza *f* medico-ospedaliera
n medische ziekenhuiskunde
d medizinische Krankenhausordnung *f*

1208 MEDICAL HOSPITALOGY
see: MEDICAL HOSPITAL KNOWLEDGE

1209 MEDICAL HOSPITAL SCIENCE
see: MEDICAL HOSPITAL KNOWLEDGE

1210 MEDICAL INFORMATION LABORATORY
f laboratoire *m* d'information médicale;
laboratoire *m* d'informatique médicale
e laboratorio *m* de información médica
i laboratorio *m* di informazione medica

n laboratorium *n* voor medische informatie
d Laboratorium *n* für medizinische Information

1211 MEDICAL INFORMATION SYSTEM
f système *m* d'information médicale;
système *m* d'informatique médicale
e sistema *m* de información médica
i sistema *m* di informazione medica
n medisch informatiesysteem *n*
d medizinisches Informationssystem *n*

1212 MEDICAL INSTRUCTION
see: MEDICAL EDUCATION

1213 MEDICAL INSTRUMENTS
f instruments *mpl* médicaux
e instrumentos *mpl* médicos
i strumenti *mpl* medici
n medische instrumenten
d medizinische Instrumente *npl*

1214 MEDICAL LABORATORY
f laboratoire *m* médical
e laboratorio *m* médico
i laboratorio *m* medico
n medisch laboratorium *n*
d medizinisches Laboratorium *n*;
ärztliches Laboratorium *n*

1215 MEDICAL LABORATORY TECHNICIAN
f technicien *m* de laboratoire médical
e técnico *m* de laboratorio médico
i tecnico *m* di laboratorio medico
n medisch laboratorium technicus
d medizinischer Laboratoriumtechniker *m*

1216 MEDICAL LAW
f droit *m* médical
e derecho *m* médico
i diritto *m* medico
n medisch recht *n*
d medizinisches Recht *n*

1217 MEDICAL LIBRARIAN
f bibliothécaire *m* médical
e bibliotecario *m* médico
i bibliotecario *m* medico
n medisch bibliothecaris
d medizinischer Bibliothekar *m*

1218 MEDICAL LIBRARY
f bibliothèque *f* médicale
e biblioteca *f* médica
i biblioteca *f* medica
n medische bibliotheek
d medizinische Bibliothek *f*

1219 MEDICAL MANPOWER;
MEDICAL PERSONNEL;
MEDICAL STAFF
f personnel *m* médical
e personal *m* médico
i personale *m* medico
n medisch personeel *n*
d ärztliches Personal *n*;
medizinisches Personal *n*

1220 MEDICAL NURSING
f soins *mpl* infirmiers médicaux
e enfermería *f* médica
i cure *fpl* infermieristiche mediche
n medische verpleging
d medizinische Pflege *f*

1221 MEDICAL ORGANIZATION
f organisation *f* médicale
e organización *f* médica
i organizzazione *f* medica
n artsenorganisatie
d ärztliche Organisation *f*

1222 MEDICAL PERSONNEL
see: MEDICAL MANPOWER

1223 MEDICAL PHOTOGRAPHER
f photographe *m* médical
e fotógrafo *m* médico
i fotografo *m* medico
n medisch fotograaf
d medizinischer Fotograf *m*

1224 MEDICAL PHOTOGRAPHY
f photographie *f* médicale
e fotografía *f* médica
i fotografia *f* medica
n medische fotografie
d medizinische Fotografie *f*

1225 MEDICAL PHOTOGRAPHY DEPARTMENT
f service *m* (département *m*) de photographie médicale
e servicio *m* (departamento *m*) de fotografía médica
i servizio *m* di fotografia medica
n afdeling medische fotografie
d medizinische Fotografieabteilung *f*

1226 MEDICAL PRACTICE
f pratique *f* médicale;
exercice *m* de la médecine
e práctica *f* de la medicina
i pratica *f* medica;
esercizio *m* della professione medica
n medische praktijk
d ärztliche Praxis *f*

1227 MEDICAL PRACTITIONER
see: DOCTOR

1228 MEDICAL PROFESSION
f profession *f* médicale
e profesión *f* médica
i professione *f* medica
n medisch beroep *n*
d medizinischer Beruf *m*

1229 MEDICAL RECORDS
see: MEDICAL ARCHIVES

1230 MEDICAL REGISTRATION
f enregistrement *m* de données médicales
e registro *m* médico
i registrazione *f* dei dati medici
n medische registratie
d medizinische Registratur *f*

1231 MEDICAL RESEARCH
f recherche *f* médicale
e investigación *f* médica
i ricerca *f* medica
n medische research
d medizinische Forschung *f*

1232 MEDICAL SCHOOL
see: MEDICAL FACULTY

1233 MEDICAL SECRET
see: MEDICAL CONFIDENTIALITY

1234 MEDICAL SECRETARY
see: MEDICAL CLERK

1235 MEDICAL SERVICE
f service *m* médical
e servicio *m* médico
i servizio *m* medico
n medische dienst
d ärztlicher Dienst *m*

1236 MEDICAL SOCIAL AID;
MEDICAL SOCIAL ASSISTANCE;
MEDICAL SOCIAL WORK
f assistance *f* médico-sociale;
aide *f* médico-sociale;
travail *m* médico-social
e asistencia *f* médico-social;
ayuda *f* médico-social;
trabajo *m* médico-social
i assistenza *f* medico-sociale;
lavoro *m* medico-sociale
n medisch-maatschappelijk werk *n*;
medisch-sociaal werk *n*
d medizinisch-soziale Fürsorge *f*

1237 MEDICAL SOCIAL ASSISTANCE
see: MEDICAL SOCIAL AID

1238 MEDICAL SOCIAL WORK
see: MEDICAL SOCIAL AID

1239 MEDICAL SOCIAL WORKER
f assistant *m* médico-social;
travailleur *m* médico-social
e asistente *m* médico-social;
trabajador *m* médico-social
i assistente *m* medico-sociale;
operatore *m* medico-sociale
n medisch-maatschappelijk werker;
medisch-sociaal werker
d Gesundheitsfürsorger *m*;
Gesundheitssozialarbeiter *m*

1240 MEDICAL SOCIOLOGIST
f sociologue *m* médical
e sociólogo *m* médico
i sociologo *m* sanitario
n medisch socioloog
d medizinischer Soziologe *m*

1241 MEDICAL SOCIOLOGY
f sociologie *f* médicale
e sociología *f* médica
i sociologia *f* sanitaria
n medische sociologie
d medizinische Soziologie *f*

1242 MEDICAL SPECIALIST
see: CONSULTANT

1243 MEDICAL SPECIALITY
f spécialité *f* médicale
e especialidad *f* médica
i specialità *f* medica
n medisch specialisme *n*
d medizinische Spezialität *f*

1244 MEDICAL SPECIALIZATION
f spécialisation *f* médicale
e especialización *f* médica
i specializzazione *f* medica
n medische specialisatie
d medizinische Spezialisierung *f*

1245 MEDICAL STAFF
see: MEDICAL MANPOWER

1246 MEDICAL STAFF LIBRARY
f bibliothèque *f* du personnel médical
e biblioteca *f* para el personal médico
i biblioteca *f* del personale medico
n bibliotheek voor het medisch personeel
d Bibliothek *f* für das ärztliche Personal

1247 MEDICAL STAFF ROOM
see: DOCTORS' QUARTER

1248 MEDICAL STATISTICS
f statistique *f* médicale
e estadística *f* médica
i statistica *f* medica
n medische statistiek
d medizinische Statistik *f*

1249 MEDICAL STUDENT;
STUDENT DOCTOR
f étudiant *m* en médecine;
étudiant *m* d'études médicales
e estudiante *m* de medicina
i studente *m* di medicina
n medisch student;
medicijnstudent;
student in de geneeskunde
d Medizinstudent *m*;
Mediziner *m*

1250 MEDICAL SUPERINTENDENT
see: CHIEF DOCTOR

1251 MEDICAL SUPERVISION
see: MEDICAL CONTROL

1252 MEDICAL-SURGICAL NURSING
f soins *mpl* infirmiers médico-chirurgicaux
e enfermería *f* médico-quirúrgica
i cure *fpl* infermieristiche medico-chirurgiche
n medisch-chirurgische verpleging
d ärztlich-chirurgische Pflege *f*

1253 MEDICAL TEACHING
see: MEDICAL EDUCATION

1254 MEDICAL TEAM
f équipe *f* médicale
e equipo *m* médico
i équipe *f* medica
n medisch team *n*
d ärztliches Team *n*

1255 MEDICAL-TECHNICAL APPARATUS
f appareils *mpl* médico-techniques
e aparatos *mpl* médico-técnicos
i apparecchi *mpl* medico-tecnici
n medisch-technische apparatuur
d medizinisch-technische Geräte *npl*

1256 MEDICAL-TECHNICAL MANPOWER;
MEDICAL-TECHNICAL PERSONNEL;
MEDICAL-TECHNICAL STAFF;
MEDICO-TECHNICAL MANPOWER;
MEDICO-TECHNICAL PERSONNEL;
MEDICO-TECHNICAL STAFF
f personnel *m* médico-technique
e personal *m* médico-técnico
i personale *m* medico-tecnico
n medisch-technisch personeel *n*
d medizinisch-technisches Personal *n*

1257 MEDICAL-TECHNICAL PERSONNEL
see: MEDICAL-TECHNICAL MANPOWER

1258 MEDICAL-TECHNICAL SERVICES;
MEDICO-TECHNICAL SERVICES
f services *mpl* médico-techniques;
services *mpl* techniques médicaux
e servicios *mpl* médico-técnicos
i servizi *mpl* tecnici medici
n medisch-technische diensten
d medizinisch-technische Dienste *mpl*

1259 MEDICAL-TECHNICAL STAFF
see: MEDICAL-TECHNICAL MANPOWER

1260 MEDICAL TECHNIQUE
see: MEDICAL ENGINEERING

1261 MEDICAL TECHNOLOGY
f technologie *f* médicale
e tecnología *f* médica
i tecnologia *f* sanitaria
n medische technologie
d medizinische Technologie *f*

1262 MEDICAL THERAPY
f thérapie *f* médicale
e terapia *f* médica
i terapia *f* medica
n medische therapie
d ärztliche Therapie *f*

1263 MEDICAL TRAINING
see: MEDICAL EDUCATION

1264 MEDICAL TREATMENT
f traitement *m* médical
e tratamiento *m* médico
i trattamento *m* medico
n medische behandeling;
geneeskundige behandeling
d ärztliche Behandlung *f*;
medizinische Behandlung *f*

1265 MEDICAL UNIT
f unité *f* médicale;
unité *f* de médecine
e unidad *f* médica;
unidad *f* de medicina
i unità *f* medica;
unità *f* di medicina
n medische eenheid
d medizinische Station *f*;
ärztliche Station *f*

1266 MEDICINAL BATH
see: MEDICAL BATH

1267 MEDICINE
see: DRUG

1268 MEDICINE TROLLEY
f chariot *m* à médicaments
e carrito *m* de medicinas
i carrello *m* per medicamenti
n medicijnwagentje *n*
d Medizinwagen *m*

1269 MEDICO-PEDAGOGICAL CENTRE (CENTER)
f centre *m* médico-pédagogique
e centro *m* médico-pedagógico
i centro *m* medico-pedagogico
n medisch opvoedkundig bureau *n*; M.O.B. *n*
d medizinisch-pädagogisches Heim *n*

1270 MEDICO-PEDAGOGICAL NURSERY
f institut *m* médico-pédagogique
e institución *f* especial de pedagogía terapéutica para niños
i istituto *m* medico-pedagogico
n inrichting voor kinderen met opvoedingsmoeilijkheden
d heilpädagogisches Kinderheim *n*

1271 MEDICO-PEDAGOGICAL REHABILITATION
f réadaptation *f* médico-pédagogique
e revalidación *f* médico-pedagógica
i riabilitazione *f* medico-pedagogica
n medisch-pedagogische revalidatie
d medizinisch-pädagogische Rehabilitation *f*

1272 MEDICO-SOCIAL SECURITY
f sécurité *f* médico-sociale
e seguridad *f* médico-social
i sicurezza *f* medico-sociale
n medisch-sociale zekerheid
d medizinisch-soziale Sicherheit *f*

1273 MEDICO-SOCIAL TEAM
f équipe *f* médico-sociale
e equipo *m* médico-social
i équipe *f* medico-sociale
n medisch-sociaal team *n*;
medisch-maatschappelijk team *n*
d medizinisch-soziales Team *n*

1274 MEDICO-SURGICAL CENTRE (CENTER)
f centre *m* médico-chirurgical
e centro *m* médico-quirúrgico
i centro *m* medico-chirurgico
n medisch-chirurgisch centrum *n*
d medizinisch-chirurgisches Zentrum *n*

1275 MEDICO-SURGICAL TEAM
f équipe *f* médico-chirurgicale
e equipo *m* médico-quirúrgico
i équipe *f* medico-chirurgica
n medisch-chirurgisch team *n*
d medizinisch-chirurgisches Team *n*

1276 MEDICO-TECHNICAL MANPOWER
see: MEDICAL-TECHNICAL MANPOWER

1277 MEDICO-TECHNICAL PERSONNEL
see: MEDICAL-TECHNICAL MANPOWER

1278 MEDICO-TECHNICAL SERVICES
see: MEDICAL-TECHNICAL SERVICES

1279 MEDICO-TECHNICAL STAFF
see: MEDICAL-TECHNICAL MANPOWER

1280 MEDIUM CARE
see: INTERMEDIATE CARE

1281 MEDIUM-SIZED HOSPITAL
f hôpital *m* de moyenne importance
e hospital *m* de tamaño medio
i ospedale *m* di media importanza
n middelgroot ziekenhuis *n*
d mittelgrosses Krankenhaus *n*;
mittleres Krankenhaus *n*

1282 MENTAL CARE;
MENTAL HEALTH CARE;
MENTAL PATIENT CARE;

PSYCHIATRIC CARE
f soins *mpl* psychiatriques;
soins *mpl* mentaux
e cuidado *m* psiquiátrico;
cuidado *m* mental;
atención *f* (asistencia *f*) psiquiátrica;
atención *f* (asistencia *f*) mental
i cure *fpl* psichiatriche
n geestelijke gezondheidszorg;
psychiatrische zorg
d psychiatrische Fürsorge *f*;
psychiatrische Versorgung *f*

1283 MENTAL DEFICIENCY;
MENTAL RETARDATION
f faiblesse *f* mentale;
déficience *f* mentale;
débilité *f* mentale
e deficiencia *f* mental;
debilidad *f* mental;
disminución *f* mental;
minusvalía *f* mental
i debolezza *f* mentale;
deficienza *f* mentale
n zwakzinnigheid
d Geistesschwäche *f*;
Schwachsinn *m*;
geistige Behinderung *f*

1284 MENTAL DISEASE;
MENTAL ILLNESS;
PSYCHIATRIC DISEASE;
PSYCHIATRIC ILLNESS
f maladie *f* mentale;
maladie *f* psychiatrique
e enfermedad *f* mental;
enfermedad *f* psiquiátrica
i malattia *f* mentale;
malattia *f* psichiatrica
n geesteziekte
d Geisteskrankheit *f*;
psychische Krankheit *f*;
Nervenkrankheit *f*

1285 MENTAL DISEASES DEPARTMENT;
MENTAL ILLNESS DEPARTMENT;
PSYCHIATRIC DEPARTMENT;
PSYCHIATRY DEPARTMENT
f service *m* (département *m*) des maladies mentales;
service *m* (département *m*) psychiatrique;
service *m* (département *m*) de psychiatrie
e servicio *m* (departamento *m*) para enfermedades mentales;
servicio *m* (departamento *m*) psiquiátrico;
servicio *m* (departamento *m*) de psiquiatría
i divisione *f* psichiatrica;
dicisione *f* di psichiatria
n psychiatrische afdeling
d psychiatrische Abteilung *f*

1286 MENTAL DISEASES DEPARTMENT (MENTAL ILLNESS DEPARTMENT, PSYCHIATRIC DEPARTMENT, PSYCHIATRY DEPARTMENT) IN A GENERAL HOSPITAL
f service *m* (département *m*) des maladies mentales dans un hôpital général;
service *m* (département *m*) psychiatrique dans un hôpital général
e servicio *m* (departamento *m*) para enfermedades mentales en un hospital general;
servicio *m* (departamento *m*) psiquiátrico en un hospital general
i divisione *f* psichiatrica in un ospedale generale
n psychiatrische afdeling in een algemeen ziekenhuis;
p.a.a.z.
d psychiatrische Abteilung *f* in einem allgemeinen Krankenhaus

1287 MENTAL DISEASES HOSPITAL;
MENTAL HOSPITAL;
MENTAL ILLNESS HOSPITAL;
PSYCHIATRIC HOSPITAL;
PSYCHIATRIC INSTITUTION;
PSYCHIATRY HOSPITAL
f hôpital *m* psychiatrique;
hôpital *m* de psychiatrie;
établissement *m* psychiatrique;
institution *f* psychiatrique;
institut *m* psychiatrique;
établissement *m* pour malades mentaux
e hospital *m* mental;
hospital *m* para enfermos mentales;
hospital *m* psiquiátrico;
institución *f* para enfermos mentales
i ospedale *m* psichiatrico;
istituto *m* psichiatrico
n psychiatrisch ziekenhuis *n*;
psychiatrisch instituut *n*;
psychiatrische inrichting
d psychiatrisches Krankenhaus *n*;
psychiatrisches Spital *n*;
psychiatrische Anstalt *f*;
psychiatrische Einrichtung *f*

1288 MENTAL DISEASES UNIT;
MENTAL ILLNESS UNIT;
PSYCHIATRIC UNIT;
PSYCHIATRY UNIT
f unité *f* des maladies mentales;
unité *f* psychiatrique;
unité *f* de psychiatrie
e unidad *f* para enfermedades mentales;
unidad *f* psiquiátrica;
unidad *f* de psiquiatría
i unità *f* psichiatrica;
unità *f* di psichiatria
n psychiatrische eenheid
d psychiatrische Station *f*

1289 MENTAL DISEASES UNIT (MENTAL ILLNESS UNIT, PSYCHIATRIC UNIT, PSYCHIATRY UNIT) IN A GENERAL HOSPITAL
f unité *f* des maladies mentales dans un hôpital général;
unité *f* psychiatrique dans un hôpital général
e unidad *f* para enfermedades mentales en un hospital general;
unidad *f* psiquiátrica en un hospital general
i unità *f* di neurologia in un ospedale generale;
unità *f* psichiatrica in un ospedale generale
n psychiatrische eenheid in een algemeen ziekenhuis
d psychiatrische Station *f* in einem allgemeinen Krankenhaus

1290 MENTAL HEALTH;
MENTAL HYGIENE
f santé *f* mentale;
hygiène *f* mentale
e salud *f* mental;
sanidad *f* mental;
higiene *f* mental
i igiene *f* mentale
n geestelijke gezondheid;
geestelijke hygiëne;

geesteshygiëne;
psychohygiëne
d geistige Gesundheit *f*;
psychische Gesundheit *f*;
Psychohygiene *f*

1291 MENTAL HEALTH CARE
see: MENTAL CARE

1292 MENTAL HEALTH CENTRE (CENTER);
PSYCHIATRIC CENTRE (CENTER)
f centre *m* de santé mentale;
centre *m* d'hygiène mentale;
centre *m* psychiatrique
e centro *m* de salud mental;
centro *m* de sanidad mental;
centro *m* psiquiátrico
i centro *m* di igiene mentale;
centro *m* psichiatrico
n centrum *n* voor geestelijke gezondheidszorg;
psychiatrisch centrum *n*
d Psychiatriezentrum *n*;
Nervenzentrum *n*

1293 MENTAL HEALTH CLINIC;
PSYCHIATRIC CLINIC
f clinique *f* de santé mentale;
clinique *f* d'hygiène mentale;
clinique *f* psychiatrique
e clínica *f* de salud mental;
clínica *f* de sanidad mental;
clínica *f* psiquiátrica
i clinica *f* di igiene mentale;
clinica *f* psichiatrica
n psychiatrische kliniek
d psychiatrische Klinik *f*

1294 MENTAL HEALTH FACILITIES;
MENTAL HEALTH SERVICES;
PSYCHIATRIC FACILITIES;
PSYCHIATRIC SERVICES;
PSYCHIATRY FACILITIES;
PSYCHIATRY SERVICES
f services *mpl* de santé mentale;
services *mpl* d'hygiène mentale;
services *mpl* psychiatriques
e servicios *mpl* de salud mental;
servicios *mpl* de sanidad mental;
servicios *mpl* sanitarios mentales;
servicios *mpl* psiquiátricos
i servizi *mpl* d'igiene mentale;
servizi *mpl* psichiatrici
n voorzieningen voor geestelijke gezondheidszorg;
psychiatrische voorzieningen
d Dienste *mpl* für geistige Gesundheit;
psychiatrische Gesundheitsdienste *mpl*

1295 MENTAL HEALTH SERVICES
see: MENTAL HEALTH FACILITIES

1296 MENTAL HOSPITAL
see: MENTAL DISEASES HOSPITAL

1297 MENTAL HYGIENE
see: MENTAL HEALTH

1298 MENTAL ILLNESS
see: MENTAL DISEASE

1299 MENTAL ILLNESS DEPARTMENT
see: MENTAL DISEASES DEPARTMENT

1300 MENTAL ILLNESS DEPARTMENT IN A GENERAL HOSPITAL
see: MENTAL DISEASES DEPARTMENT IN A GENERAL HOSPITAL

1301 MENTAL ILLNESS HOSPITAL
see: MENTAL DISEASES HOSPITAL

1302 MENTAL ILLNESS UNIT
see: MENTAL DISEASES UNIT

1303 MENTAL ILLNESS UNIT IN A GENERAL HOSPITAL
see: MENTAL DISEASES UNIT IN A GENERAL HOSPITAL

1304 MENTALLY HANDICAPPED DEPARTMENT;
MENTAL SUBNORMALITY DEPARTMENT
f service *m* (département *m*) pour handicapés mentaux
e servicio *m* (departamento *m*) para débiles mentales
i servizio *m* per l'assistenza degli handicappati mentali
n afdeling voor geestelijk gehandicapten
d Abteilung *f* für geistig Behinderte

1305 MENTALLY HANDICAPPED UNIT;
MENTAL SUBNORMALITY UNIT
f unité *f* pour handicapés mentaux
e unidad *f* para débiles mentales
i unità *f* per l'assistenza degli handicappati mentali
n eenheid voor geestelijk gehandicapten
d Station *f* für geistig Behinderte

1306 MENTAL PATIENT;
PSYCHIATRIC PATIENT
f malade *m* (patient *m*) mental;
malade *m* (patient *m*) psychiatrique
e paciente *m* (enfermo *m*) mental;
paciente *m* (enfermo *m*) psiquiátrico
i malato *m* mentale;
malato *m* di mente;
malato *m* psichiatrico
n geesteszieke;
psychiatrische patiënt
d Geisteskranker *m*;
Nervenkranker *m*;
psychiatrischer Patient *m*;
psychisch Kranker *m*

1307 MENTAL PATIENT CARE
see: MENTAL CARE

1308 MENTAL RETARDATION
see: MENTAL DEFICIENCY

1309 MENTAL SUBNORMALITY DEPARTMENT
see: MENTALLY HANDICAPPED DEPARTMENT

1310 MENTAL SUBNORMALITY UNIT
see: MENTALLY HANDICAPPED UNIT

1311 METABOLIC DEPARTMENT
f service *m* (département *m*) du métabolisme
e servicio *m* (departamento *m*) de metabolismo
i servizio *m* dis-endocrino - dis-metabolico
n afdeling voor stofwisselingsonderzoek
d Grundumsatzabteilung *f*

1312 METABOLIC DISEASE
f maladie *f* du métabolisme
e enfermedad *f* metabólica
i malattia *f* metabolica
n stofwisselingsziekte
d Stoffwechselkrankheit *f*

1313 MICROBIOLOGICAL LABORATORY;
MICROBIOLOGY LABORATORY
f laboratoire *m* de microbiologie
e laboratorio *m* de microbiología
i laboratorio *m* di microbiologia
n microbiologisch laboratorium *n*
d Laboratorium *n* für Mikrobiologie

1314 MICROBIOLOGIST
f microbiologiste *m*
e microbiólogo *m*
i microbiologo *m*
n microbioloog
d Mikrobiologe *m*

1315 MICROBIOLOGY
f microbiologie *f*
e microbiología *f*
i microbiologia *f*
n microbiologie
d Mikrobiologie *f*

1316 MICROBIOLOGY LABORATORY
see: MICROBIOLOGICAL LABORATORY

1317 MIDDLE CARE
see: INTERMEDIATE CARE

1318 MIDWIFE;
OBSTETRICIAN
f accoucheuse *f*;
sage-femme *f*
e partera *f*;
comadre *f*;
comadrona *f*;
matrona *f*
i levatrice *f*;
ostetrica *f*
n vroedvrouw;
verloskundige
d Hebamme *f*;
Geburtshelferin *f*

1319 MIDWIFERY;
OBSTETRICS
f obstétrique *f*
e obstetricia *f*;
tocología *f*
i ostetricia *f*
n verloskunde;
obstetrie
d Geburtshilfe *f*;
Frauenheilkunde *f*;
Obstetrik *f*

1320 MILITARY HOSPITAL
see: ARMED FORCES HOSPITAL

1321 MILITARY MEDICINE
f médecine *f* militaire
e medicina *f* militar
i medicina *f* militare
n militaire geneeskunde
d Militärmedizin *f*

1322 MILITARY PHARMACIST
f pharmacien *m* militaire
e farmacéutico *m* militar;
boticario *m* militar
i farmacista *m* militare
n militaire apotheker
d Militärapotheker *m*

1323 MILITARY PHYSICIAN
f médecin *m* militaire
e médico *m* militar
i medico *m* militare
n militaire arts
d Militärarzt *m*

1324 MINIMAL CARE
see: LOW CARE

1325 MINIMAL CARE DEPARTMENT
see: LOW CARE DEPARTMENT

1326 MINIMAL CARE PATIENT
see: LOW CARE PATIENT

1327 MINIMAL CARE UNIT
see: LOW CARE UNIT

1328 MIXED UNIT
f unité *f* mixte
e unidad *f* mixta
i unità *f* mista
n gemengde eenheid
d gemischte Station *f*

1329 MOBILE CLINIC
f clinique *f* mobile
e clínica *f* móvil
i clinica *f* mobile
n rijdende kliniek
d fahrbare Klinik *f*

1330 MORBIDITY;
SICK-RATE
f morbidité *f*
e morbididad *f*;
morbilidad *f*
i morbilità *f*
n ziektecijfer *n*;
morbiditeit
d Morbidität *f*

1331 MORBIDITY STATISTICS
f statistique *f* de morbidité
e estadística *f* de morbididad
i statistica *f* della morbilità
n morbiditeitsstatistiek
d Morbiditätsstatistik *f*

1332 MORBID MATTER
f agent *m* pathogène;
matière *f* morbifique
e agente *m* patógeno
i agente *m* patogeno
n ziektestof
d Krankheitsstoff *m*

1333 MORBID SYMPTOM
f symptôme *m*
e síntoma *m* de enfermedad
i sintomo *m*
n ziektesymptoom *n*;
ziekteverschijnsel *n*
d Krankheitssymptom *n*;
Krankheitserscheinung *f*

1334 MORGUE;
MORTUARY
f morgue *f* ;
chambre *f* mortuaire;
dépositoire *m*

e mortuorio *m*
i camera *f* mortuaria;
obitorio *m*
n mortuarium *n*
d Leichenhalle *f*

1335 MORTALITY
see: DEATH RATE

1336 MORTALITY STATISTICS
f statistique *f* de mortalité
e estadística *f* de mortalidad
i statistica *f* della mortalità
n mortaliteitsstatistiek
d Mortalitätsstatistik *f*

1337 MORTUARY
see: MORGUE

1338 MUD BATH
f bain *m* de boue
e baño *m* de fango
i bagno *m* di fango
n modderbad *n*
d Schlammbad *n*

1339 MUNICIPAL HEALTH CARE FACILITIES;
MUNICIPAL HEALTH CARE SERVICES;
MUNICIPAL HEALTH FACILITIES;
MUNICIPAL HEALTH SERVICES
f services *mpl* sanitaires municipaux
e servicios *mpl* sanitarios municipales
i servizi *mpl* sanitari municipali
n gemeentelijke gezondheidsdiensten;
G.G.D.
d kommunale Gesundheitsdienste *mpl*

1340 MUNICIPAL HEALTH CARE SERVICES
see: MUNICIPAL HEALTH CARE FACILITIES

1341 MUNICIPAL HEALTH FACILITIES
see: MUNICIPAL HEALTH CARE FACILITIES

1342 MUNICIPAL HEALTH SERVICES
see: MUNICIPAL HEALTH CARE FACILITIES

1343 MUNICIPAL HOSPITAL
f hôpital *m* municipal
e hospital *m* municipal
i ospedale *m* municipale
n gemeenteziekenhuis *n*
d Gemeindekrankenhaus *n*

1344 MUSIC THERAPY
f thérapie *f* de musique
e terapia *f* de música
i psicoterapia *f* musicale
n muziektherapie
d Musiktherapie *f*

N

1345 NARCOSIS
f narcose *f*
e narcosis *f*
i narcosi *f*
n narcose
d Narkose *f*

1346 NATALITY
see: BIRTH-RATE

1347 NATALITY STATISTICS
f statistique *f* de natalité
e estadística *f* de natalidad
i statistica *f* della natalità
n geboortestatistiek
d Geburtenstatistik *f*

1348 NATIONAL HEALTH SERVICE
f service *m* national de santé
e servicio *m* sanitario nacional;
servicio *m* nacional de salud
i servizio *m* sanitario nazionale
n nationale gezondheidszorg
d nationaler Gesundheitsdienst *m*

1349 NECROPSY
see: AUTOPSY

1350 NECROSCOPY
see: AUTOPSY

1351 NEONATAL CARE;
NEWBORN CARE
f soins *mpl* aux nouveau-nés
e cuidado *m* (atención *f*) de recién nacidos
i cura *f* dei neonati
n verzorging van pas geboren baby's
d Neugeborenenpflege *f*

1352 NEONATAL MEDICINE
f médecine *f* néonatale
e medicina *f* neonatal
i medicina *f* neonatale
n zuigelingengeneeskunde
d Neugeborenenmedizin *f*

1353 NEONATAL ROOM;
NEWBORN NURSERY
f salle *f* pour nouveau-nés;
pouponnière *f*;
pouponnat *m*
e sala *f* para recién nacidos;
guardería *f* de lactantes
i sala *f* per neonati
n babykamer;
wiegenkamer
d Neugeborenenzimmer *n*;
Neugeborenenraum *m*;
Säuglingszimmer *n*

1354 NEPHROLOGY
f néphrologie *f*
e nefrología *f*
i nefrologia *f*
n nefrologie
d Nephrologie *f*

1355 NERVOUS DISEASES CLINIC;
NEUROLOGICAL CLINIC;
NEUROLOGY CLINIC
f clinique *f* des maladies neurologiques;
clinique *f* neurologique;
clinique *f* de neurologie
e clínica *f* para enfermedades nerviosas;
clínica *f* neurológica;
clínica *f* de neurología
i clinica *f* neurologica;
clinica *f* di neurologia
n neurologische kliniek;
kliniek voor zenuwziekten
d neurologische Klinik *f*;
Nervenklinik *f*

1356 NERVOUS DISEASES DEPARTMENT;
NEUROLOGICAL DEPARTMENT;
NEUROLOGY DEPARTMENT
f service *m* (département *m*) des maladies neurologiques;
service *m* (département *m*) neurologique;
service *m* (département *m*) de neurologie
e servicio *m* (departamento *m*) para enfermedades nerviosas;
servicio *m* (departamento *m*) neurológico;
servicio *m* (departamento *m*) de neurología
i divisione *f* neurologica;
divisione *f* di neurologia
n neurologische afdeling;
afdeling voor zenuwziekten
d neurologische Abteilung *f*;
Nervenabteilung *f*

1357 NERVOUS DISEASES HOSPITAL;
NEUROLOGICAL HOSPITAL;
NEUROLOGY HOSPITAL
f hôpital *m* des maladies neurologiques;
hôpital *m* neurologique;
hôpital *m* de neurologie
e hospital *m* para enfermedades nerviosas;
hospital *m* neurológico;
hospital *m* de neurología
i ospedale *m* neurologico;
ospedale *m* di neurologia
n neurologisch ziekenhuis *n*
d neurologisches Krankenhaus *n*;
Nervenheilanstalt *f*

1358 NERVOUS DISEASES UNIT;
NEUROLOGICAL UNIT;
NEUROLOGY UNIT
f unité *f* des maladies neurologiques;
unité *f* neurologique;
unité *f* de neurologie
e unidad *f* para enfermedades nerviosas;
unidad *f* neurológica;
unidad *f* de neurología
i unità *f* neurologica;
unità *f* di neurologia
n neurologische eenheid;
eenheid voor zenuwziekten
d neurologische Station *f*

1359 NEUROLOGICAL CLINIC
see: NERVOUS DISEASES CLINIC

1360 NEUROLOGICAL DEPARTMENT
see: NERVOUS DISEASES DEPARTMENT

1361 NEUROLOGICAL HOSPITAL
see: NERVOUS DISEASES HOSPITAL

1362 NEUROLOGICAL SURGERY;
NEUROSURGERY
f neurochirurgie *f*
e neurocirugía *f*
i neurochirurgia *f*
n neurochirurgie
d Neurochirurgie *f*

1363 NEUROLOGICAL UNIT
see: NERVOUS DISEASES UNIT

1364 NEUROLOGIST
f neurologiste *m*;
neurologue *m*
e neurólogo *m*
i neurologo *m*
n neuroloog;
zenuwarts
d Neurologe *m*;
Nervenarzt *m*

1365 NEUROLOGY
f neurologie *f*
e neurología *f*
i neurologia *f*
n neurologie
d Neurologie *f*

1366 NEUROLOGY CLINIC
see: NERVOUS DISEASES CLINIC

1367 NEUROLOGY DEPARTMENT
see: NERVOUS DISEASES DEPARTMENT

1368 NEUROLOGY HOSPITAL
see: NERVOUS DISEASES HOSPITAL

1369 NEUROLOGY UNIT
see: NERVOUS DISEASES UNIT

1370 NEUROPSYCHIATRIC CLINIC
f clinique *f* neuropsychiatrique;
clinique *f* de neuropsychiatrie
e clínica *f* neuropsiquiátrica;
clínica *f* de neuropsiquiatría
i clinica *f* neuropsichiatrica;
clinica *f* di neuropsichiatria
n neuropsychiatrische kliniek
d neurologisch-psychiatrische Klinik *f*

1371 NEUROPSYCHIATRIC HOSPITAL
f hôpital *m* neuropsychiatrique;
hôpital *m* de neuropsychiatrie
e hospital *m* neuropsiquiátrico;
hospital *m* de neuropsiquiatría
i ospedale *m* neuropsichiatrico;
ospedale *m* di neuropsichiatria
n neuropsychiatrisch ziekenhuis *n*
d neurologisch-psychiatrische Anstalt *f*

1372 NEUROPSYCHIATRIST
f neuropsychiatre *m*
e neuropsiquiatra *m*
i neuropsichiatra *m*
n neuropsychiater
d Neuropsychiater *m*

1373 NEUROPSYCHIATRY
f neuropsychiatrie *f*
e neuropsiquiatría *f*
i neuropsichiatria *f*
n neuropsychiatrie
d Neuropsychiatrie *f*

1374 NEUROSURGEON
f neurochirurgien *m*
e neurocirujano *m*
i neurochirurgo *m*
n neurochirurg
d Neurochirurg *m*

1375 NEUROSURGERY
see: NEUROLOGICAL SURGERY

1376 NEUROSURGERY CLINIC;
NEUROSURGICAL CLINIC
f clinique *f* neurochirurgicale;
clinique *f* de neurochirurgie
e clínica *f* neuroquirúrgica;
clínica *f* de neurocirugía
i clinica *f* neurochirurgica;
clinica *f* di neurochirurgia
n neurochirurgische kliniek
d neurochirurgische Klinik *f*

1377 NEUROSURGERY DEPARTMENT;
NEUROSURGICAL DEPARTMENT
f service *m* (département *m*) neurochirurgical;
service *m* (département *m*) de neurochirurgie
e servicio *m* (departamento *m*) neuroquirúrgico;
servicio *m* (departamento *m*) de neurocirugía
i divisione *f* neurochirurgica;
divisione *f* di neurochirurgia
n neurochirurgische afdeling
d neurochirurgische Abteilung *f*

1378 NEUROSURGERY HOSPITAL;
NEUROSURGICAL HOSPITAL
f hôpital *m* neurochirurgical;
hôpital *m* de neurochirurgie
e hospital *m* neuroquirúrgico;
hospital *m* de neurocirugía
i ospedale *m* neurochirurgico;
ospedale *m* di neurochirurgia
n neurochirurgisch ziekenhuis *n*
d neurochirurgisches Krankenhaus *n*

1379 NEUROSURGERY UNIT;
NEUROSURGICAL UNIT
f unité *f* neurochirurgicale;
unité *f* de neurochirurgie
e unidad *f* neuroquirúrgica;
unidad *f* de neurocirugía
i unità *f* neurochirurgica;
unità *f* di neurochirurgia
n neurochirurgische eenheid
d neurochirurgische Station *f*

1380 NEUROSURGICAL CLINIC
see: NEUROSURGERY CLINIC

1381 NEUROSURGICAL DEPARTMENT
see: NEUROSURGERY DEPARTMENT

1382 NEUROSURGICAL HOSPITAL
see: NEUROSURGERY HOSPITAL

1383 NEUROSURGICAL UNIT
see: NEUROSURGERY UNIT

1384 NEWBORN BASSINET
f lit *m* pour nouveau-nés
e cuna *f* para recién nacidos
i letto *m* per neonati
n wieg voor zuigelingen
d Bettchen *n* für Neugeborene

1385 NEWBORN CARE
see: NEONATAL CARE

1386 NEWBORN NURSERY
see: NEONATAL ROOM

1387 NIGHT CARE
f soins *mpl* de nuit
e cuidado *m* nocturno;
atención *f* (asistencia *f*) nocturna
i cure *fpl* notturne
n nachtverzorging
d Nachtversorgung *f*

1388 NIGHT CLINIC
f clinique *f* de nuit
e clínica *f* nocturna;
clínica *f* de noche
i clinica *f* notturna
n nachtkliniek
d Nachtklinik *f*

1389 NIGHT HOSPITAL
f hôpital *m* de nuit
e hospital *m* nocturno;
hospital *m* de noche
i ospedale *m* notturno
n nachtziekenhuis *n*
d Nachtkrankenhaus *n*;
Nachtspital *n*

1390 NIGHT HOSPITALIZATION
f hospitalisation *f* de nuit
e hospitalización *f* nocturna;
hospitalización *f* de noche
i ospedalizzazione *f* notturna
n nachthospitalisatie
d Nachtversorgung *f* in einem Krankenhaus

1391 NIGHT LABORATORY
f laboratoire *m* de nuit
e laboratorio *m* nocturno;
laboratorio *m* de noche
i laboratorio *m* notturno
n nachtlaboratorium *n*
d Nachtlaboratorium *n*

1392 NIGHT NURSE
f infirmière *f* de nuit;
veilleuse *f* de nuit
e enfermera *f* de noche
i infermiera *f* vigilatrice notturna
n nachtzuster
d Nachtschwester *f*

1393 NIGHT NURSING
f soins *mpl* infirmiers de nuit
e enfermería *f* nocturna;
enfermería *f* de noche
i cure *fpl* infermieristiche notturne
n nachtverpleging
d Nachtpflege *f*

1394 NIGHT PATIENT
f malade *m* (patient *m*) de nuit
e paciente *m* (enfermo *m*) nocturno;
paciente *m* (enfermo *m*) de noche
i malato *m* notturno
n nachtpatiënt
d Nachtpatient *m*

1395 NIGHT PHARMACY
f pharmacie *f* de nuit
e farmacia *f* de noche;
botica *f* de noche
i farmacia *f* notturna
n nachtapotheek
d Nachtapotheke *f*

1396 NIGHT PSYCHIATRIC TREATMENT
f traitement *m* psychiatrique de nuit
e tratamiento *m* psiquiátrico nocturno;
tratamiento *m* psiquiátrico de noche
i trattamento *m* psichiatrico notturno
n psychiatrische nachtbehandeling
d psychiatrische Nachtbehandlung *f*

1397 NIGHT TREATMENT
f traitement *m* de nuit
e tratamiento *m* nocturno;
tratamiento *m* de noche
i trattamento *m* notturno
n nachtbehandeling
d Nachtbehandlung *f*

1398 NON-ACADEMIC HOSPITAL;
NON-TEACHING HOSPITAL;
NON-UNIVERSITY HOSPITAL
f hôpital *m* non-académique;
centre *m* hospitalier non-universitaire;
hôpital *m* non-universitaire
e hospital *m* no-académico;
hospital *m* no-universitario;
hospital *m* no-docente
i ospedale *m* non universitario
n niet-academisch ziekenhuis *n*;
niet-universitair ziekenhuis *n*
d nicht-akademisches Krankenhaus *n*;
Nicht-Universitätskrankenhaus *n*;
Nicht-Unterrichtskrankenhaus *n*;
Nicht-Ausbildungskrankenhaus *n*;
Nicht-Lehrkrankenhaus *n*

1399 NON-AMBULANT INPATIENT
f malade *m* (patient *m*) hospitalisé non-ambulant
e paciente *m* (enfermo *m*) hospitalizado no-ambulante
i malato *m* ospedalizzato non in grado di alzarsi
n niet-ambulante klinische patiënt
d nicht-ambulanter stationärer Patient *m*

1400 NON-AMBULANT OUTPATIENT
f malade *m* (patient *m*) externe non-ambulant
e paciente *m* (enfermo *m*) externo no-ambulante
i malato *m* esterno non in grado di alzarsi
n niet-ambulante poliklinische patiënt
d nicht-ambulanter Poliklinikpatient *m*

1401 NON-AMBULANT PATIENT
see: BEDRIDDEN PATIENT

1402 NON-INSTITUTIONAL CARE
see: EXTRAMURAL CARE

1403 NON-INSTITUTIONAL FACILITIES
see: EXTRAMURAL FACILITIES

1404 NON-INSTITUTIONAL HEALTH CARE
see: EXTRAMURAL HEALTH CARE

1405 NON-INSTITUTIONAL HEALTH FACILITIES
see: EXTRAMURAL HEALTH FACILITIES

1406 NON-MEDICAL MANPOWER;
NON-MEDICAL PERSONNEL;
NON-MEDICAL STAFF
f personnel *m* non-médical
e personal *m* no-médico
i personale *m* non medico
n niet-medisch personeel *n*
d nicht-medizinisches Personal *n*;
nicht-ärztliches Personal *n*

1407 NON-MEDICAL PERSONNEL
see: NON-MEDICAL MANPOWER

1408 NON-MEDICAL SERVICE
f service *m* non-médical
e servicio *m* no-médico
i servizio *m* non medico
n niet-medische dienst
d nicht-ärztlicher Dienst *m*

1409 NON-MEDICAL STAFF
see: NON-MEDICAL MANPOWER

1410 NON-NURSE MANPOWER;
NON-NURSE PERSONNEL;
NON-NURSING STAFF
f personnel *m* non-infirmier
e personal *m* no de enfermería
i personale *m* non infermieristico
n niet-verpleegkundig personeel *n*
d nicht-pflegerisches Personal *n*

1411 NON-NURSE PERSONNEL
see: NON-NURSE MANPOWER

1412 NON-NURSING STAFF
see: NON-NURSE MANPOWER

1413 NON-PROFIT HOSPITAL;
NON-PROFIT MAKING HOSPITAL
f hôpital *m* sans but lucratif;
hôpital *m* à but non lucratif;
établissement *m* hospitalier à but non lucratif
e hospital *m* sin fines de lucro;
hospital *m* no montado como negocio
i ospedale *m* senza fini lucrativi
n ziekenhuis *n* zonder winstoogmerk;
non-profit ziekenhuis *n*
d gemeinnütziges Krankenhaus *n*

1414 NON-PROFIT MAKING HOSPITAL
see: NON-PROFIT HOSPITAL

1415 NON-TEACHING HOSPITAL
see: NON-ACADEMIC HOSPITAL

1416 NON-UNIVERSITY HOSPITAL
see: NON-ACADEMIC HOSPITAL

1417 NORMAL CARE
see: INTERMEDIATE CARE

1418 NUCLEAR DIAGNOSIS
f diagnose *f* nucléaire
e diagnosis *f* nuclear
i diagnosi *f* nucleare
n nucleaire diagnose
d Nukliddiagnose *f*

1419 NUCLEAR MEDICINE
f médecine *f* nucléaire
e medicina *f* nuclear
i medicina *f* nucleare
n nucleaire geneeskunde
d Nuklearmedizin *f*;
Kernmedizin *f*

1420 NUCLEAR MEDICINE DEPARTMENT
f service *m* (département *m*) de médecine nucléaire
e servicio *m* (departamento *m*) de medicina nuclear
i servizio *m* di medicina nucleare
n afdeling nucleaire geneeskunde
d nuklearmedizinische Abteilung *f*

1421 NUCLEAR THERAPY
f thérapie *f* nucléaire
e terapia *f* nuclear
i terapia *f* nucleare
n nucleaire therapie
d Nuklidtherapie *f*;
Nukleartherapie *f*

1422 NUMBER OF BEDS OCCUPIED
f nombre *m* des lits occupés
e número *m* de camas ocupadas
i numero *m* dei letti occupati
n aantal *n* bezette bedden
d Zahl *f* der belegten Betten

1423 NUMBER OF BEDS PER 1000 INHABITANTS
f nombre *m* des lits par 1000 habitants
e número *m* de camas por 1.000 habitantes
i posti-letto *mpl* per 1000 abitanti;
numero *m* di letti per 1000 abitanti
n aantal *n* bedden per 1000 inwoners
d Bettenzahl *f* pro 1000 Einwohner

1424 NURSE
see: ATTENDANT

1425 NURSE AIDE
see: AIDE

1426 NURSE-ANESTHETIST
see: ANESTHESIA NURSE

1427 NURSE CALL SYSTEM;
NURSES CALL SYSTEM
f système *m* d'appel des infirmières
e sistema *m* de llamada de las enfermeras
i sistema *m* di chiamata delle infermiere
n zusteroproepsysteem *n*
d Schwesternrufsystem *n*

1428 NURSE CLOTHING
f vêtements *mpl* d'infirmière
e vestidos *mpl* de enfermeras
i vestiti *mpl* d'infermiera
n verpleegsterskleding
d Schwesternkleidung *f*;
Schwesterntracht *f*

1429 NURSE EDUCATION;
NURSE TRAINING;
NURSING EDUCATION;
NURSING TRAINING
f enseignement *m* infirmier;
formation *f* infirmière

e formación *f* de enfermeras;
educación *f* de enfermeras;
enseñanza *f* para enfermeras
i formazione *f* del personale sanitario ausiliario
n verpleegkundige opleiding;
verpleegkundig onderwijs *n*;
opleiding van verplegenden
d Krankenpflegeausbildung *f*;
Krankenpfleger(innen)ausbildung *f*;
Pfleger(innen)ausbildung *f*;
Krankenschwesternausbildung *f*;
Schwesternausbildung *f*

1430 NURSE MANPOWER;
NURSE PERSONNEL;
NURSING MANPOWER;
NURSING PERSONNEL;
NURSING STAFF
f personnel *m* infirmier
e personal *m* de enfermería
i personale *m* infermieristico
n verpleegkundig personeel *n*;
verplegend personeel *n*
d Krankenpflegepersonal *n*;
Pflegepersonal *n*;
pflegerisches Personal *n*

1431 NURSE/PATIENT COMMUNICATION SYSTEM
f système *m* de communication infirmière/malade
e sistema *m* de comunicación enfermera/paciente
i sistema *m* di communicazione infermiera/malato
n communicatiesysteem *n* verplegende/patiënt
d Kommunikationssystem *n* Krankenpflegerin/Patient

1432 NURSE/PATIENT RELATION
f relation *f* infirmière/malade
e relación *f* enfermera/paciente
i relazione *f* infermiera/malato
n relatie verplegende/patiënt
d Verhältnis *n* Krankenpflegerin/Patient

1433 NURSE PERSONNEL
see: NURSE MANPOWER

1434 NURSE RECRUITMENT
f recrutement *m* d'infirmières
e reclutamiento *m* de enfermeras
i assunzione *f* delle infermiere
n werving van verpleegkundigen
d Werbung *f* von Krankenpflegerinnen

1435 NURSES' ASSOCIATION
f association *f* d'infirmières
e asociación *f* de enfermeras
i associazione *f* d'infermiere
n vereniging van verpleegkundigen
d Schwesternverein *m*;
Schwesternverband *m*

1436 NURSES CALL SYSTEM
see: NURSE CALL SYSTEM

1437 NURSES' DESK;
NURSES' STATION
f poste *m* d'infirmières
e puesto *m* de enfermeras;
estación *f* de enfermeras
i sala *f* delle infermiere
n verpleegsterspost;
zusterpost
d Krankenschwesternstation *f*;
Schwesternstation *f*

1438 NURSES' FLAT
f appartement *m* des infirmières
e piso *m* para las enfermeras
i alloggio *m* delle infermiere
n verpleegstersflat
d Schwesternappartement *n*

1439 NURSES' HOME;
NURSES' RESIDENCE
f habitation *f* des infirmières;
foyer *m* des infirmières
e vivienda *f* de las enfermeras
i alloggio *m* delle infermiere
n verpleegsters(te)huis *n*;
zusterhuis *n*;
internaat *n* voor verpleegsters
d Schwestern(wohn)heim *n*;
Schwestern(wohn)haus *n*;
Schwesterngebäude *n*

1440 NURSES' HOUSING
f logement *m* pour les infirmières
e alojamiento *m* para las enfermeras
i alloggio *m* delle infermiere
n huisvesting voor verplegenden;
zusterhuisvesting
d Schwesternwohnungen *fpl*

1441 NURSES' OFFICE;
NURSES' ROOM
f chambre *f* des infirmières
e cuarto *m* para las enfermeras
i camera *f* riservata alle infermiere
n verpleegsterskamer;
zusterkamer
d Krankenpflegerinnenzimmer *n*;
Schwesternzimmer *n*

1442 NURSES' PREPARATORY TRAINING SCHOOL;
PRELIMINARY NURSES' SCHOOL;
PRELIMINARY NURSE TRAINING SCHOOL;
PRELIMINARY NURSING SCHOOL;
PRE-NURSING SCHOOL
f école *f* préparatoire aux études d'infirmière;
école *f* préparatoire d'infirmières
e escuela *f* preparatoria para enfermeras
i scuola *f* preparatoria agli studi d'infermiera
n voorbereidende verpleegstersschool
d Krankenpflegevorschule *f*;
Pflegevorschule *f*;
Schwesternvorschule *f*

1443 NURSES' RESIDENCE
see: NURSES' HOME

1444 NURSES' ROOM
see: NURSES' OFFICE

1445 NURSES' SCHOOL;
NURSES' TRAINING SCHOOL;
NURSING SCHOOL;
SCHOOL FOR NURSES;
SCHOOL FOR NURSING;
SCHOOL OF NURSING;
TRAINING SCHOOL FOR NURSES
f école *f* infirmière;
école *f* d'infirmières;
école *f* d'enseignement infirmier
e escuela *f* de enfermería;
escuela *f* de (para) enfermeras;
escuela *f* de enseñanza para enfermeras

i scuola *f* per infermiere;
scuola *f* di formazione professionale per infermiere
n verpleegstersschool;
school voor verplegenden
d Krankenpflegeschule *f*;
Pflegerinnenschule *f*;
Schwesternschule *f*;
Schule *f* für Schwesternausbildung

1446 NURSES' STATION
see: NURSES' DESK

1447 NURSES' TRAINING SCHOOL
see: NURSES' SCHOOL

1448 NURSES' TUTOR;
NURSE TUTOR
f monitrice *f*;
infirmière-monitrice *f*
e tutora *f*;
enfermera *f* tutora
i vigilatrice *f*;
infermiera-vigilatrice *f*
n mentrix
d Mentrix *f*

1449 NURSES' UNIFORM
f uniforme *m* d'infirmière
e uniforme *m* de enfermeras
i uniforme *f* d'infermiera
n verpleegstersuniform *n*
d Schwesternuniform *f*

1450 NURSE TRAINING
see: NURSE EDUCATION

1451 NURSE TUTOR
see: NURSES' TUTOR

1452 NURSING;
NURSING CARE
f soins *mpl* infirmiers
e enfermería *f*;
cuidado *m* enfermero;
atención *f* (asistencia *f*) enfermera;
cuidado *m* (atención *f*, asistencia *f*) de enfermería
i cure *fpl* infermieristiche;
assistenza *f* infermieristica
n (zieken)verpleging;
verpleegkundige zorg
d Pflegearbeit *f*;
Krankenpflege *f*;
pflegerische Versorgung *f*

1453 NURSING ARTICLES
f articles *mpl* pour les soins aux malades
e artículos *mpl* de enfermería
i articoli *mpl* impiegati per la cura degli ammalati
n verplegingsartikelen
d Krankenpflegeartikel *mpl*

1454 NURSING ASSISTANT
see: AIDE

1455 NURSING AUDIT
f contrôle *m* de la qualité des soins infirmiers
e auditoria *f* enfermera;
evaluación *f* del cuidado enfermero
i controllo *m* della qualità delle cure infermieristiche
n nursing audit;
kwaliteitsmeting van de verpleegkundige zorg
d Qualitätskontrole *f* der pflegerischen Versorgung

1456 NURSING AUXILIARY
see: AIDE

1457 NURSING CARE
see: NURSING

1458 NURSING CARE SYSTEM
f système *m* de soins infirmiers
e sistema *m* de cuidado enfermero
i sistema *m* di cure infermieristiche
n verpleegsysteem *n*
d Pflegesystem *n*

1459 NURSING CENTRE (CENTER)
see: CHRONIC CARE INSTITUTION

1460 NURSING COURSE;
NURSING EDUCATION COURSE
f cours *m* de formation infirmière
e curso *m* de enfermera;
curso *m* de formación de enfermeras
i corso *m* per l'addestramento del personale infermieristico
n verpleegkundige cursus
d Krankenpflegekurs(us) *m*

1461 NURSING DEPARTMENT;
NURSING SERVICE DEPARTMENT
f service *m* (département *m*) infirmier;
service *m* (département *m*) de soins infirmiers
e servicio *m* (departamento *m*) de enfermería;
servicio *m* (departamento *m*) de enfermeras
i servizio *m* infermieristico
n verpleegafdeling
d Pflegeabteilung *f*

1462 NURSING EDUCATION
see: NURSE EDUCATION

1463 NURSING EDUCATION COURSE
see: NURSING COURSE

1464 NURSING HISTORY
see: HISTORY OF NURSING

1465 NURSING HOME
CHRONIC CARE INSTITUTION

1466 NURSING JOURNAL
f revue *f* des infirmières
e revista *f* enfermera;
revista *f* para enfermeras
i rivista *f* per le infermiere
n verpleegkundig tijdschrift *n*
d Krankenpflegezeitschrift *f*;
Pflegezeitschrift *f*

1467 NURSING LIBRARY
f bibliothèque *f* pour infirmières
e biblioteca *f* enfermera;
biblioteca *f* para enfermeras
i biblioteca *f* per infermiere
n verpleegkundige bibliotheek
d Bibliothek *f* für Krankenpflegerinnen

1468 NURSING MANPOWER
see: NURSE MANPOWER

1469 NURSING PERSONNEL
see: NURSE MANPOWER

1470 NURSING PROFESSION
f profession *f* infirmière;

profession *f* d'infirmière
e profesión *f* enfermera;
profesión *f* de enfermera
i professione *f* d'infermiera
n verpleegkundig beroep *n*
d Krankenpflegeberuf *m*;
Pflegeberuf *m*

1471 NURSING RESEARCH
f recherche *f* en soins infirmiers
e investigación *f* enfermera;
investigación *f* en enfermería
i ricerca *f* nel campo dell' assistenza infermieristica
n verpleegkundige research;
verpleegkundig onderzoekswerk *n*
d Forschung *f* in der Krankenpflege

1472 NURSING SCHOOL
see: NURSES' SCHOOL

1473 NURSING SCIENCE;
SCIENCE OF NURSING
f sciences *fpl* infirmières
e ciencia *f* enfermera
i scienze *fpl* infermieristiche
n verpleegkunde
d Krankenpflege *f*

1474 NURSING SERVICE
f service *m* infirmier
e servicio *m* de enfermería
i servizio *m* infermieristico
n verplegingsdienst
d Krankenpflegedienst *m*;
Pflegedienst *m*;
Pflegewesen *n*

1475 NURSING SERVICE DEPARTMENT
see: NURSING DEPARTMENT

1476 NURSING SHORTAGE;
SHORTAGE OF NURSES
f manque *m* d'infirmières
e falta *f* de enfermeras
i mancanza *f* d'infermiere
n verpleegsterstekort *n*
d Schwesternmangel *m*

1477 NURSING STAFF
see: NURSE MANPOWER

1478 NURSING STUDENT;
PUPIL NURSE;
STUDENT NURSE
f élève-infirmière *f*;
apprentie-infirmière *f*
e enfermera *f* alumna;
alumna *f* de enfermera
i allieva *f* infermiera
n leerling-verpleegkundige;
leerling-verplegende;
leerling-verpleegster
d Pflegeschülerin *f*;
Krankenpflegeschülerin *f*;
Lernschwester *f*

1479 NURSING STUDIES
f études *fpl* d'infirmière
e estudios *mpl* de enfermera
i studi *mpl* d'infermiera
n verpleegkundige studies
d Pflegestudien *npl*

1480 NURSING TEAM
f équipe *f* soignante
e equipo *m* de enfermeras
i équipe *f* curante
n verpleegkundig team *n*
d Pflegeteam *n*

1481 NURSING TRAINING
see: NURSE EDUCATION

1482 NURSING TREATMENT
f traitement *m* infirmier
e tratamiento *m* enfermero
i trattamento *m* infermieristico
n verpleegkundige behandeling
d Pflegebehandlung *f*

1483 NURSING UNIT
see: INPATIENT CARE UNIT

1484 NUTRITIONAL HYGIENE
see: FOOD HYGIENE

1485 NUTRITION SERVICE
see: FOOD SERVICE

O

1486 OBLIGATORY HEALTH CARE INSURANCE
see: COMPULSORY HEALTH CARE INSURANCE

1487 OBLIGATORY HEALTH INSURANCE
see: COMPULSORY HEALTH CARE INSURANCE

1488 OBSERVATION DEPARTMENT
f service *m* (département *m*) d'observation
e servicio *m* (departamento *m*) de observación
i servizio *m* d'osservazione
n observatie-afdeling
d Beobachtungsabteilung *f*

1489 OBSERVATION ROOM
f chambre *f* d'observation
e sala *f* de observación
i camera *f* d'osservazione
n observatieruimte
d Beobachtungsraum *m*

1490 OBSERVATION UNIT
f unité *f* d'observation
e unidad *f* de observación
i unità *f* d'osservazione
n observatie-eenheid
d Beobachtungsstation *f*

1491 OBSTETRIC CARE
f soins *mpl* obstétricaux
e cuidado *m* obstétrico;
atención *f* obstétrica;
cuidado *m* (atención *f*) de obstetricia
i cure *fpl* ostetriche
n verloskundige zorg
d Geburtshilfe *f*

1492 OBSTETRIC CLINIC
see: MATERNITY CLINIC

1493 OBSTETRIC DEPARTMENT
see: MATERNITY DEPARTMENT

1494 OBSTETRIC HOSPITAL
see: MATERNITY HOSPITAL

1495 OBSTETRICIAN
see: MIDWIFE

1496 OBSTETRIC NURSE
see: MATERNITY NURSE

1497 OBSTETRIC NURSING
see: MATERNITY NURSING

1498 OBSTETRICS
see: MIDWIFERY

1499 OBSTETRIC UNIT
see: MATERNITY UNIT

1500 OCCUPATIONAL DISEASE
see: INDUSTRIAL DISEASE

1501 OCCUPATIONAL HEALTH SERVICE
see: INDUSTRIAL HEALTH SERVICE

1502 OCCUPATIONAL HYGIENE
see: INDUSTRIAL HYGIENE

1503 OCCUPATIONAL MEDICAL SERVICE
see: INDUSTRIAL HEALTH SERVICE

1504 OCCUPATIONAL MEDICINE
see: INDUSTRIAL MEDICINE

1505 OCCUPATIONAL NURSING
see: INDUSTRIAL NURSING

1506 OCCUPATIONAL PHYSICIAN
see: FACTORY PHYSICIAN

1507 OCCUPATIONAL THERAP(EUT)IST
f thérapeute *m* occupationnel
e terapeuta *m* ocupacional
i terapeuta *m* occupazionale;
terapista *m* occupazionale
n bezigheidstherapeut
d Beschäftigungstherapeut *m*

1508 OCCUPATIONAL THERAPY
f thérapie *f* occupationnelle;
thérapie *f* par l'occupation
e terapia *f* ocupacional
i terapia *f* occupazionale
n bezigheidstherapie
d Beschäftigungstherapie *f*

1509 OCCUPATIONAL THERAPY DEPARTMENT
f service *m* (département *m*) de thérapie occupationnelle
e servicio *m* (departamento *m*) de terapia ocupacional
i servizio *m* di terapia occupazionale
n bezigheidstherapeutische afdeling
d Abteilung *f* für Beschäftigungstherapie

1510 OCULIST
see: EYE SPECIALIST

1511 OLD AGE HOME
see: GERIATRIC HOME

1512 OLD PEOPLE CARE
see: CARE OF OLD PEOPLE

1513 OLD PEOPLE HOME
see: GERIATRIC HOME

1514 OPEN CLINIC
f clinique *f* ouverte
e clínica *f* abierta
i clinica *f* aperta
n open kliniek
d Belegklinik *f*

1515 OPEN HOSPITAL
f hôpital *m* ouvert
e hospital *m* abierto
i ospedale *m* aperto
n open ziekenhuis *n*
d Belegkrankenhaus *n*

1516 OPERATING BLOCK;
OPERATING DEPARTMENT;
OPERATING SUITE;
SURGERY BLOCK;
SURGERY DEPARTMENT;
SURGERY SUITE;
SURGICAL BLOCK;
SURGICAL DEPARTMENT;
SURGICAL SUITE
f bloc *m* opératoire;
bloc *m* chirurgical;
service *m* (département *m*) chirurgical;
service *m* (département *m*) de chirurgie
e servicio *m* (departamento *m*) quirúrgico;
servicio *m* (departamento *m*) de cirugía;
servicio *m* (departamento *m*) de operaciones;
bloque *m* quirúrgico
i blocco *m* operatorio
n operatie-afdeling;
chirurgische afdeling
d Operationsabteilung *f*;
chirurgische Abteilung *f*;
Operationstrakt *m*;
Operationsblock *m*;
Operationsbereich *m*

1517 OPERATING DEPARTMENT
see: OPERATING BLOCK

1518 OPERATING ROOM;
OPERATING THEATRE;
OPERATIONS ROOM
f salle *f* d'opérations;
salle *f* opératoire;
théâtre *m* d'opérations;
théâtre *m* opératoire
e sala *f* operatoria;
sala *f* de operaciones;
sala *f* quirúrgica;
sala *f* de cirugía;
teatro *m* operatorio;
teatro *m* de operaciones;
quirófano *m*
i sala *f* operatoria;
sala *f* d'operazioni;
anfiteatro *m* chirurgico
n operatiekamer
d Operationsraum *m*;
Operationssaal *m*

1519 OPERATING ROOM CLOTHING;
OPERATING THEATRE CLOTHING;
OPERATION CLOTHING;
OPERATIONS ROOM CLOTHING;
SURGICAL CLOTHING;
THEATRE CLOTHING
f vêtements *mpl* opératoires;
vêtements *mpl* pour salles d'opérations
e vestidos *mpl* para la sala operatoria
i vestiti *mpl* per sale operatorie
n operatie(kamer)kleding
d Operationskleidung *f*

1520 OPERATING ROOM LINEN;
OPERATING THEATRE LINEN;
OPERATION LINEN;
OPERATIONS ROOM LINEN;
SURGICAL LINEN;
THEATRE LINEN
f linge *m* opératoire;
linge *m* pour salles d'opérations
e ropa *f* para la sala operatoria
i biancheria *f* per sale operatorie
n operatie(kamer)linnen *n*
d Operationswäsche *f*;
Operationsleinwand *f*

1521 OPERATING ROOM NURSE;
OPERATING THEATRE NURSE;
THEATRE NURSE
f infirmière *f* de salle d'opérations
e enfermera *f* de sala operatoria
i infermiera *f* di sala operatoria
n operatieverpleegkundige;
o.k.-verpleegkundige
d Operationsschwester *f*

1522 OPERATING ROOM NURSING;
OPERATING THEATRE NURSING;
THEATRE NURSING
f soins *mpl* infirmiers de salle d'opérations
e enfermería *f* de sala operatoria
i cure *fpl* infermieristiche in sala operatoria
n operatieverpleging;
o.k.-verpleging
d Operationspflege *f*

1523 OPERATING ROOM SISTER;
OPERATING THEATRE SISTER;
THEATRE SISTER
f infirmière-chef *f* de salle d'opérations
e enfermera *f* jefe de sala operatoria
i infermiera-capo *f* di sala operatoria
n hoofdverpleegkundige op de operatiekamer;
hoofdverpleegkundige op de o.k.
d Operationsoberschwester *f*

1524 OPERATING SUITE
see: OPERATING BLOCK

1525 OPERATING TABLE
f table *f* d'opérations
e mesa *f* de operaciones
i tavola *f* operatoria
n operatietafel
d Operationstisch *m*

1526 OPERATING THEATRE
see: OPERATING ROOM

1527 OPERATING THEATRE CLOTHING
see: OPERATING ROOM CLOTHING

1528 OPERATING THEATRE LINEN
see: OPERATING ROOM LINEN

1529 OPERATING THEATRE NURSE
see: OPERATING ROOM NURSE

1530 OPERATING THEATRE NURSING
see: OPERATING ROOM NURSUNG

1531 OPERATING THEATRE SISTER
see: OPERATING ROOM SISTER

1532 OPERATION;
SURGICAL OPERATION
f opération *f*
e operación *f*
i operazione *f*
n operatie
d Operation *f*

1533 OPERATION CLOTHING
see: OPERATING ROOM CLOTHING

1534 OPERATION LAMP
f lampe *f* pour opérations
e lámpara *f* de operaciones
i lampada *f* per sala operatoria
n operatielamp
d Operationslampe *f*

1535 OPERATION LINEN
see: OPERATING ROOM LINEN

1536 OPERATION MASK
f masque *m* d'opérations
e máscara *f* de operaciones
i maschera *f* operatoria
n operatiemasker *n*
d Operationsmaske *f*

1537 OPERATIONS ROOM
see: OPERATING ROOM

1538 OPERATIONS ROOM CLOTHING
see: OPERATING ROOM CLOTHING

1539 OPERATIONS ROOM LINEN
see: OPERATING ROOM LINEN

1540 OPHTHALMIC CLINIC
see: EYE CLINIC

1541 OPHTHALMIC DEPARTMENT
see: EYE DEPARTMENT

1542 OPHTHALMIC HOSPITAL
see: EYE HOSPITAL

1543 OPHTHALMIC SURGERY
see: EYE SURGERY

1544 OPHTHALMIC UNIT
see: EYE UNIT

1545 OPHTHALMOLOGIST
see: EYE SPECIALIST

1546 OPHTHALMOLOGY
f ophtalmologie *f*
e oftalmología *f*
i oftalmologia *f*;
oculistica *f*
n oogheelkunde
d Augenheilkunde *f*

1547 OPHTHALMOLOGY CLINIC
see: EYE CLINIC

1548 OPHTHALMOLOGY DEPARTMENT
see: EYE DEPARTMENT

1549 OPHTHALMOLOGY HOSPITAL
see: EYE HOSPITAL

1550 OPHTHALMOLOGY UNIT
see: EYE UNIT

1551 OPTICIAN
f opticien *m*
e óptico *m*
i ottico *m*
n opticien
d Optiker *m*

1552 OPTOMETRY
f optométrie *f*
e optometría *f*
i optometria *f*
n optometrie
d Optometrie *f*

1553 ORAL HYGIENE
f hygiène *f* orale
e higiene *f* oral
i igiene *f* orale
n mondhygiëne
d Mundhygiene *f*

1554 ORGAN TRANSPLANT(ATION)
f greffe *f* d'organes;
transplantation *f* d'organes
e trasplante *m* de órganos
i trapianto *m* d'organi
n orgaantransplantatie
d Organübertragung *f*;
Organtransplantation *f*

1555 ORTHODONTICS
f orthodontie *f*
e ortodontía *f*
i ortodonzia *f*
n orthodontie
d Orthodontie *f*

1556 ORTHODONTICS DEPARTMENT
f service *m* (département *m*) orthodontique;
service *m* (département *m*) d'orthodontie
e servicio *m* (departamento *m*) ortodóntico;
servicio *m* (departamento *m*) de ortodontía
i divisione *f* di odontoiatria
n orthodontische afdeling
d orthodontische Abteilung *f*

1557 ORTHODONTICS HOSPITAL
f hôpital *m* orthodontique;
hôpital *m* d'orthodontie
e hospital *m* ortodóntico;
hospital *m* de ortodontía
i ospedale *m* odontoiatrico
n orthodontisch ziekenhuis *n*
d orthodontisches Krankenhaus *n*

1558 ORTHODONTICS UNIT
f unité *f* orthodontique;
unité *f* d'orthodontie
e unidad *f* ortodóntica;
unidad *f* de ortodontía
i unità *f* di odontoiatria
n orthodontische eenheid
d orthodontische Station *f*

1559 ORTHOPEDIC CARE
f soins *mpl* orthopédiques
e cuidado *m* ortopédico;
asistencia *f* ortopédica
i cure *fpl* ortopediche
n orthopedische (ver)zorg(ing)
d orthopädische Versorgung *f*

1560 ORTHOPEDIC CLINIC
f clinique *f* orthopédique;
clinique *f* d'orthopédie
e clínica *f* ortopédica;
clínica *f* de ortopedia

i clinica *f* ortopedica
n orthopedische kliniek
d orthopädische Klinik *f*

1561 ORTHOPEDIC DEPARTMENT
f service *m* (département *m*) orthopédique;
service *m* (département *m*) d'orthopédie
e servicio *m* (departamento *m*) ortopédico;
servicio *m* (departamento *m*) de ortopedia
i divisione *f* ortopedica
n orthopedische afdeling
d orthopädische Abteilung *f*

1562 ORTHOPEDIC HOSPITAL
f hôpital *m* orthopédique;
hôpital *m* d'orthopédie
e hospital *m* ortopédico;
hospital *m* de ortopedia
i ospedale *m* ortopedico
n orthopedisch ziekenhuis *n*
d orthopädisches Krankenhaus *n*

1563 ORTHOPEDIC NURSING
f soins *mpl* infirmiers orthopédiques
e cuidado *m* enfermero ortopédico
i cure *fpl* infermieristiche ortopediche
n orthopedische verpleging
d orthopädische Pflege *f*

1564 ORTHOPEDICS
f orthopédie *f*
e ortopedia *f*
i ortopedia *f*
n orthopedie
d Orthopädie *f*

1565 ORTHOPEDIC SURGERY
f chirurgie *f* orthopédique
e cirugía *f* ortopédica
i chirurgia *f* ortopedica
n orthopedische chirurgie
d orthopädische Chirurgie *f*

1566 ORTHOPEDIC UNIT
f unité *f* orthopédique;
unité *f* d'orthopédie
e unidad *f* ortopédica;
unidad *f* de ortopedia
i unità *f* ortopedica
n orthopedische eenheid
d orthopädische Station *f*

1567 ORTHOPEDIST
f orthopédiste *m*
e ortopedista *m*;
ortopédico *m*
i ortopedico *m*
n orthopedist
d Orthopädist *m*

1568 OTORHINOLARYNGOLOGY
f oto-rhino-laryngologie *f*
e otorrinolaringología *f*
i otorinolaringologia *f*;
otorinolaringoiatria *f*
n keel- neus- en oorheelkunde
d Hals- Nasen- und Ohrenheilkunde *f*

1569 OUTPATIENT
see: AMBULATORY PATIENT

1570 OUTPATIENT CARE
see: AMBULANT CARE

1571 OUTPATIENT CARE INSTITUTION;
OUTPATIENT CLINIC;
POLYCLINIC
f consultations *fpl* externes;
polyclinique *f*
e policlínica *f*;
ambulatorio *m*
i poliambulatori *mpl*;
consultorio *m*
n polikliniek
d Poliklinik *f*;
Ambulatorium *n*

1572 OUTPATIENT CLINIC
see: OUTPATIENT CARE INSTITUTION

1573 OUTPATIENT CONSULTATION
see: AMBULATORY CONSULTATION

1574 OUTPATIENT DEPARTMENT;
POLYCLINICAL DEPARTMENT
f service *m* (département *m*) de consultations externes;
service *m* (département *m*) de traitement ambulatoire
e servicio *m* (departamento *m*) de consultas externas;
servicio *m* (departamento *m*) de pacientes externos;
servicio *m* (departamento *m*) de visitas externas
i servizio *m* di consultazioni
n poliklinische afdeling
d ambulante Abteilung *f*;
Abteilung *f* für ambulante Patienten (Behandlung)

1575 OUTPATIENT HEALTH CARE
see: AMBULANT HEALTH CARE

1576 OUTPATIENT PSYCHIATRIC CARE
f soins *mpl* psychiatriques ambulatoires
e cuidado *m* psiquiátrico ambulatorio;
atención *f* psichiátrica ambulatoria
i cure *fpl* psichiatriche ambulatoriali
n poliklinische psychiatrische zorg;
ambulatorische psychiatrische zorg
d ambulante psychiatrische Fürsorge *f*;
ambulante psychiatrische Versorgung *f*

1577 OUTPATIENT SERVICES
see: AMBULATORY CARE SERVICES

1578 OUTPATIENT SURGERY
f chirurgie *f* ambulatoire
e cirugía *f* ambulatoria
i chirurgia *f* ambulatoriale
n poliklinische chirurgie
d ambulante Chirurgie *f*

1579 OUTPATIENT TREATMENT
see: AMBULATORY TREATMENT

1580 OXYGEN CHAMBER
f chambre *f* d'oxygène
e cámara *f* de oxígeno
i camera *f* per la somministrazione di ossigeno
n zuurstofkamer
d Sauerstoffraum *m*

1581 OXYGEN DISTRIBUTION
f distribution *f* d'oxygène
e distribución *f* de oxígeno
i distribuzione *f* di ossigeno
n zuurstofvoorziening
d Sauerstoffversorgung *f*

1582 OXYGEN THERAPY
f oxygénothérapie *f*
e oxigenoterapia *f*
i ossigenoterapia *f*
n zuurstoftherapie
d Sauerstofftherapie *f*

1583 OXYGEN THERAPY DEPARTMENT
f service *m* (département *m*) d'oxygénothérapie
e servicio *m* (departamento *m*) de oxigenoterapia
i servizio *m* d'ossigenoterapia
n zuurstoftherapie-afdeling
d Sauerstofftherapie-Abteilung *f*

P

1584 PANEL DOCTOR
f médecin *m* de caisse
e médico *m* de la caja
i medico *m* della mutua
n fondsdokter
d Kassenarzt *m*

1585 PARAMEDICAL EDUCATION; PARAMEDICAL INSTRUCTION; PARAMEDICAL TEACHING; PARAMEDICAL TRAINING
f formation *f* paramédicale; enseignement *m* paramédical
e educación *f* paramédica; enseñanza *f* paramédica
i formazione *f* paramedica
n paramedische opleiding; paramedisch onderwijs *n*
d paramedizinische Ausbildung *f*; paramedizinischer Unterricht *m*

1586 PARAMEDICAL INSTRUCTION
see: PARAMEDICAL EDUCATION

1587 PARAMEDICAL MANPOWER; PARAMEDICAL PERSONNEL; PARAMEDICAL STAFF
f personnel *m* paramédical
e personal *m* paramédico
i personale *m* paramedico
n paramedisch personeel *n*
d paramedizinisches Personal *n*

1588 PARAMEDICAL PERSONNEL
see: PARAMEDICAL MANPOWER

1589 PARAMEDICAL PROFESSION
f profession *f* paramédicale
e profesión *f* paramédica
i professione *f* paramedica
n paramedisch beroep *n*
d paramedizinischer Beruf *m*

1590 PARAMEDICAL STAFF
see: PARAMEDICAL MANPOWER

1591 PARAMEDICAL TEACHING
see: PARAMEDICAL EDUCATION

1592 PARAMEDICAL TRAINING
see: PARAMEDICAL EDUCATION

1593 PARAPLEGIC CENTRE (CENTER)
f centre *m* pour paraplégiques
e centro *m* para parapléjicos
i centro *m* paraplegici
n centrum *n* voor paraplegie patiënten
d Paraplegikerzentrum *n*

1594 PARASITOLOGIST
f parasitologiste *m*; parasitologue *m*
e parasitólogo *m*
i parassitologo *m*
n parasitoloog
d Parasitologe *m*

1595 PARASITOLOGY
f parasitologie *f*
e parasitología *f*
i parassitologia *f*
n parasitologie
d Parasitologie *f*

1596 PARENTS' ROOM
f chambre *f* des parents
e sala *f* para los padres
i sala *f* dei parenti
n ouderkamer
d Elternraum *m*

1597 PART-TIME DOCTOR; PART-TIME MEDICAL PRACTITIONER; PART-TIME PHYSICIAN
f médecin *m* à temps partiel
e médico *m* a tiempo parcial
i medico *m* a metà tempo; medico *m* a tempo definito
n part-time arts
d Part Time Arzt *m*; Belegarzt *m*

1598 PART-TIME HOSPITALIZATION
f hospitalisation *f* partielle
e hospitalización *f* parcial
i ospedalizzazione *f* parziale
n partiële hospitalisatie
d Part Time Krankenhauseinweisung *f*

1599 PART-TIME HOSPITAL TREATMENT
f traitement *m* hospitalier partiel
e tratamiento *m* hospitalario parcial
i trattamento *m* ospedaliero parziale
n partiële ziekenhuisbehandeling
d Part Time Krankenhausbehandlung *f*

1600 PART-TIME MEDICAL PRACTITIONER
see: PART-TIME DOCTOR

1601 PART-TIME NURSE
f infirmière *f* à temps partiel
e enfermera *f* a tiempo parcial
i infermiera *f* a metà tempo; infermiera *f* a tempo definito
n part- time verpleegster
d Part Time Krankenpflegerin *f*

1602 PART-TIME PHYSICIAN
see: PART-TIME DOCTOR

1603 PATHOGRAPHY
f nosographie *f*
e patografía *f*
i nosografia *f*
n ziektebeschrijving
d Krankheitsbeschreibung *f*

1604 PATHOLOGICAL DEPARTMENT; PATHOLOGY DEPARTMENT
f service *m* (département *m*) pathologique; service *m* (département *m*) de pathologie
e servicio *m* (departamento *m*) patológico; servicio *m* (departamento *m*) de patología

i servizio *m* di istologia e di anatomia patologica
n pathologische afdeling
d pathologische Abteilung *f*

1605 PATHOLOGICAL LABORATORY;
PATHOLOGY LABORATORY
f laboratoire *m* pathologique;
laboratoire *m* de pathologie
e laboratorio *m* patológico;
laboratorio *m* de patología
i laboratorio *m* di istologia e di anatomia patologica
n pathologisch laboratorium *n*
d pathologisches Laboratorium *n*

1606 PATHOLOGIST
f pathologiste *m*
e patólogo *m*
i anatomo-patologo *m*
n patholoog
d Pathologe *m*

1607 PATHOLOGY
f pathologie *f*
e patología *f*
i patologia *f*
n pathologie
d Pathologie *f*

1608 PATHOLOGY DEPARTMENT
see: PATHOLOGICAL DEPARTMENT

1609 PATHOLOGY LABORATORY
see: PATHOLOGICAL LABORATORY

1610 PATIENT
f malade *m*;
patient *m*
e paciente *m*;
enfermo *m*
i malato *m*;
paziente *m*
n patiënt;
zieke
d Patient *m*;
Kranker *m*

1611 PATIENT ADMINISTRATION
f administration *f* des malades
e administración *f* de los pacientes
i amministrazione *f* relativa ai malati
n patiëntenadministratie
d patientengebundene Verwaltung *f*;
Patientenverwaltung *f*

1612 PATIENT CARE
f soins *mpl* aux (des) malades (patients)
e cuidado *m* del paciente (enfermo);
atención *f* del paciente (enfermo)
i cura *f* dei malati (pazienti);
assistenza *f* dei malati (pazienti)
n patiëntenzorg;
ziekenzorg
d Patientenversorgung *f*;
Krankenversorgung *f*;
Patientenbetreuung *f*;
Krankenbetreuung *f*

1613 PATIENT CARE UNIT
see: INPATIENT CARE UNIT

1614 PATIENT CHAIR
f chaise *f* pour malades
e sillón *m* de paciente
i sedia *f* per malati
n patiëntenstoel
d Patientenstuhl *m*

1615 PATIENT CLASSIFICATION
f classification *f* des malades
e clasificación *f* de los pacientes
i classificazione *f* dei malati
n patiëntenclassificatie
d Patientenklassifikation *f*

1616 PATIENT DATA
f données *fpl* des malades
e datos *mpl* de los pacientes
i dati *mpl* sui malati
n patiëntengegevens
d Patientendaten *npl*

1617 PATIENT DATA BANK
f banque *f* de données des malades
e banco *m* de datos de los paciente
i banca *f* dei dati sui malati
n bank voor patiëntengegevens
d Patientendatenbank *f*

1618 PATIENT DATA SYSTEM
f système *m* de données des malades
e sistema *m* de datos de los pacientes
i sistema *m* dei dati sui malati
n systeem *n* voor patiëntengegevens
d Patientendatensystem *n*

1619 PATIENT DAY
see: DAY OF CARE

1620 PATIENT EDUCATION
f éducation *f* du malade
e educación *f* del paciente
i educazione *f* del malato
n patiëntenopvoeding
d Patientenerziehung *f*

1621 PATIENT FLOW;
PATIENT TURNOVER
f mouvement *m* des malades;
rotation *f* des malades
e movimiento *m* de los pacientes;
ingresos *mpl* de los pacientes
i movimento *m* dei malati;
rotazione *f* dei malati
n patiëntenverloop *n*;
patiëntendoorstroming
d Patientendurchgang *m*;
Patientenbewegung *f*

1622 PATIENT HANDLING
f gestion *f* des malades
e tratamiento *m* de los pacientes
i gestione *f* dei malati
n patiëntenbehandeling
d Patientenbehandlung *f*

1623 PATIENT MONITORING;
PATIENT SUPERVISION
f surveillance *f* des malades
e vigilancia *f* de los pacientes;
control *m* de los pacientes
i sorveglianza *f* dei malati;
monitoraggio *m* dei malati
n patiëntenbewaking
d Patientenüberwachung *f*

1624 PATIENT MONITORING SYSTEM;
PATIENT SUPERVISION SYSTEM
f système *m* de surveillance des malades
e sistema *m* de vigilancia de los pacientes
i sistema *m* di sorveglianza dei malati
n patiëntenbewakingssysteem *n*
d Patientenüberwachungssystem *n*

1625 PATIENT/NURSE CALL SYSTEM
f système *m* d'appel malade/infirmière
e sistema *m* de llamada paciente/enfermera
i sistema *m* di chiamata malato/infermiera
n patiënt/zusteroproepsysteem *n*
d Patient/Schwesterrufanlage *f*

1626 PATIENT NURSING
f soins *mpl* infirmiers aux malades
e cuidado *m* enfermero de los pacientes
i cure *fpl* infermieristiche dei malati
n patiëntenverpleging
d Patientenpflege *f*

1627 PATIENT RECEPTION
f réception *f* des malades
e recepción *f* de los pacientes
i accettazione *f* dei malati
n opvang van de patiënt
d Patientenaufnahme *f*

1628 PATIENT REGISTRATION
f enregistrement *m* des malades
e registro *m* de los pacientes
i registrazione *f* dei malati
n patiëntenregistratie
d Eintragung *f* der Patienten

1629 PATIENT ROOM;
PATIENTS' ROOM;
SICK ROOM;
WARD ROOM
f chambre *f* de malade;
salle *f* de malade;
chambre *f* d'hospitalisation
e cuarto *m* del paciente;
habitación *f* del paciente;
pieza *f* del paciente
i camera *f* per malati;
camera *f* d'ospedale
n patiëntenkamer;
ziekenkamer;
verpleegkamer
d Patientenzimmer *n*;
Krankenzimmer *n*;
Krankenhauszimmer *n*

1630 PATIENTS' CLOTHES
f vêtements *mpl* des malades
e vestidos *mpl* de los pacientes
i vestiti *mpl* dei malati;
abbigliamento *m* per malati
n patiëntenkleding
d Patientenkleidung *f*

1631 PATIENTS' COMPLAINT
f plainte *f* des malades
e queja *f* de los pacientes
i reclamo *m* dei malati
n klacht van patiënten
d Beschwerde *f* der Patienten

1632 PATIENTS' COUNCIL
f conseil *m* des malades
e consejo *m* de los pacientes
i consiglio *m* dei malati
n patiëntenraad
d Patientenrat *m*

1633 PATIENTS' ELEVATOR;
PATIENTS' LIFT
f ascenseur *m* pour malades;
élévateur *m* pour malades
e ascensor *m* para pacientes
i ascensore *m* per il trasporto dei malati
n patiëntenlift
d Patientenaufzug *m*;
Patientenheber *m*

1634 PATIENTS' LIBRARY
f bibliothèque *f* pour les malades
e biblioteca *f* para los pacientes
i biblioteca *f* dei malati
n patiëntenbibliotheek
d Patientenbücherei *f*;
Patientenbibliothek *f*

1635 PATIENTS' LIFT
see: PATIENTS' ELEVATOR

1636 PATIENTS' PROPERTY
f propriété *f* des malades
e propiedad *f* de los pacientes
i proprietà *f* dei malati
n patiënteneigendom *n*
d Patienteneigentum *n*

1637 PATIENTS' RECREATION
f récréation *f* des malades
e recreo *m* de los pacientes
i ricreazione *f* dei malati
n ontspanning van de patiënt
d Patientenerholung *f*

1638 PATIENTS' RIGHT
f droit *m* du malade
e derecho *m* del paciente
i diritto *m* del malato
n patiëntenrecht *n*
d Patientenrecht *n*

1639 PATIENTS' ROOM
see: PATIENT ROOM

1640 PATIENTS' SHOP
f boutique *f* pour les malades
e tienda *f* para los pacientes
i negozio *m* per gli ammalati
n patiëntenwinkeltje *n*
d Patientenladen *m*

1641 PATIENT SUPERVISION
see: PATIENT MONITORING

1642 PATIENT SUPERVISION SYSTEM
see: PATIENT MONITORING SYSTEM

1643 PATIENT TRANSFER
f transfer *m* du malade
e traslado *m* del paciente
i trasferimento *m* dei malati
n overplaatsing van de patiënt
d Überbringung *f* des Patienten

1644 PATIENT TRANSPORT(ATION)
see: HEALTH TRANSPORT

1645 PATIENT TURNOVER
see: PATIENT FLOW

1646 PATIENT UNIT
see: INPATIENT CARE UNIT

1647 PATIENT WEIGHING MACHINE
f bascule *f* pour malades
e báscula *f* para pacientes
i bilancia *m* per malati
n patiëntenweegschaal
d Patientenwaage *f*

1648 PATIENT WHEEL CHAIR
f fauteuil *m* à roulettes pour malades
e silla *f* ambulante para pacientes; butaca *f* de ruedas para pacientes; sillón *m* de ruedas para pacientes
i poltrona *f* con le rotelle per malati
n rolstoel voor patiënten
d Patientenfahrstuhl *m*

1649 PEDIATRIC CARE
f soins *mpl* pédiatriques
e cuidado *m* pediátrico
i cure *fpl* pediatriche
n kinderverzorging
d Kinderversorgung *f*

1650 PEDIATRIC CLINIC
see: CHILDREN'S CLINIC

1651 PEDIATRIC DEPARTMENT
see: CHILDREN'S DEPARTMENT

1652 PEDIATRIC HEALTH CARE
see: CHILDREN'S HEALTH CARE

1653 PEDIATRIC HOSPITAL
see: CHILDREN'S HOSPITAL

1654 PEDIATRICIAN
see: CHILD HEALTH SPECIALIST

1655 PEDIATRIC NURSING
f soins *mpl* infirmiers pédiatriques
e enfermería *f* pediátrica
i cure *fpl* infermieristiche pediatriche
n kinderverpleging
d Kinderpflege *f*

1656 PEDIATRICS
f pédiatrie *f*
e pediatría *f*
i pediatria *f*
n pediatrie; kindergeneeskunde
d Pädiatrie *f*; Kinderheilkunde *f*

1657 PEDIATRIC UNIT
see: CHILDREN'S UNIT

1658 PERINATAL MORBIDITY
f morbidité *f* périnatale
e morbididad *f* perinatal; morbilidad *f* perinatal
i morbilità *f* perinatale
n perinatale morbiditeit
d perinatale Morbidität *f*

1659 PERINATAL MORTALITY
f mortalité *f* périnatale
e mortalidad *f* perinatal
i mortalità *f* perinatale
n perinatale mortaliteit
d perinatale Mortalität *f*

1660 PERINATAL UNIT
f unité *f* périnatale
e unidad *f* perinatal
i unità *f* perinatale
n perinatale eenheid
d perinatale Station *f*

1661 PERIPHERAL HOSPITAL
f hôpital *m* périphérique
e hospital *m* periférico
i ospedale *m* periferico
n perifeer ziekenhuis *n*
d peripherisches Krankenhaus *n*

1662 PERSONAL HYGIENE
f hygiène *f* personnelle
e higiene *f* personal
i igiene *f* personale
n persoonlijke hygiëne
d persönliche Hygiene *f*

1663 PERSONNEL HEALTH CARE; STAFF HEALTH CARE
f soins *mpl* sanitaires du personnel; soins *mpl* de santé du personnel
e cuidado *m* sanitario del personal; atención *f* sanitaria del personal
i assistenza *f* sanitaria del personale
n personeelsgezondheidszorg
d Personalgesundheitspflege *f*

1664 PERSONNEL HEALTH SERVICE; STAFF HEALTH SERVICE
f service *m* sanitaire du personnel
e servicio *m* sanitario del personal
i servizio *m* sanitario del personale
n personeelsgezondheidsdienst
d Personalgesundheitsdienst *m*

1665 PERSONNEL/PATIENT RATE; PERSONNEL/PATIENT RATIO; STAFF/PATIENT RATE; STAFF/PATIENT RATIO
f proportion *f* personnel/malades
e proporción *f* personal/pacientes
i rapporto *m* personale/pazienti
n verhouding personeel/patiënten
d Verhältnis *n* Personal/Patienten

1666 PERSONNEL/PATIENT RATIO
see: PERSONNEL/PATIENT RATE

1667 PEST CONTROL
f lutte *f* contre la peste
e lucha *f* contra la peste
i lotta *f* contro la peste
n pestbestrijding
d Pestbekämpfung *f*

1668 PHARMACEUTICAL DEPARTMENT; PHARMACY DEPARTMENT
f service *m* (département *m*) pharmaceutique

e servicio *m* (departamento *m*) farmacéutico
i farmacia *f* interna
n farmaceutische afdeling
d pharmazeutische Abteilung *f*

1669 PHARMACEUTICAL LABORATORY
f laboratoire *m* pharmaceutique
e laboratorio *m* farmacéutico
i laboratorio *m* farmaceutico
n farmaceutisch laboratorium *n*
d pharmazeutisches Laboratorium *n*

1670 PHARMACEUTICAL RESEARCH
f recherche *f* pharmaceutique
e investigación *f* farmacéutica
i ricerca *f* farmaceutica
n farmaceutisch onderzoek *n*
d pharmazeutische Forschung *f*

1671 PHARMACIST
f pharmacien *m*
e farmacéutico *m*;
boticario *m*
i farmacista *m*
n apotheker
d Apotheker *m*

1672 PHARMACOLOGIST
f pharmacologiste *m*
e farmacólogo *m*
i farmacologo *m*
n farmacoloog
d Pharmakologe *m*

1673 PHARMACOLOGY
f pharmacologie *f*
e farmacología *f*
i farmacologia *f*
n farmacologie
d Pharmakologie *f*

1674 PHARMACOTHERAPY
f pharmacothérapie *f*
e farmacoterapia *f*
i farmacoterapia *f*
n farmacotherapie
d Pharmakotherapie *f*

1675 PHARMACY
f pharmacie *f*
e farmacia *f*;
botica *f*
i farmacia *f*
n apotheek
d Apotheke *f*

1676 PHARMACY DEPARTMENT
see: PHARMACEUTICAL DEPARTMENT

1677 PHOTOGRAPHY DEPARTMENT
f service *m* (département *m*) de photographie
e servicio *m* (departamento *m*) de fotografía
i servizio *m* di fotografia
n foto-afdeling
d Fotoabteilung *f*

1678 PHOTOGRAPHY LABORATORY
f laboratoire *m* de photographie
e laboratorio *m* de fotografía
i laboratorio *m* di fotografia
n fotolaboratorium *n*
d Fotolaboratorium *n*

1679 PHOTOGRAPHY MANPOWER;
PHOTOGRAPHY PERSONNEL;
PHOTOGRAPHY STAFF
f personnel *m* de photographie
e personal *m* de fotografía
i personale *m* addetto alla fotografia
n fotografiepersoneel *n*
d Fotopersonal *n*

1680 PHOTOGRAPHY PERSONNEL
see: PHOTOGRAPHY MANPOWER

1681 PHOTOGRAPHY STAFF
see: PHOTOGRAPHY MANPOWER

1682 PHYSICAL CULTURE;
PHYSICAL EDUCATION
f culture *f* physique;
éducation *f* physique
e instrucción *f* física;
educación *f* física
i cultura *f* fisica
n lichamelijke opvoeding
d Körpererziehung *f*

1683 PHYSICAL DISEASE;
PHYSICAL ILLNESS;
SOMATIC DISEASE;
SOMATIC ILLNESS
f maladie *f* physique;
maladie *f* somatique
e enfermedad *f* física;
enfermedad *f* somática
i malattia *f* fisica;
malattia *f* somatica
n lichamelijke ziekte;
somatische ziekte
d körperliche Krankheit *f*;
somatische Krankheit *f*

1684 PHYSICAL EDUCATION
see: PHYSICAL CULTURE

1685 PHYSICAL EXAMINATION
f examen *m* fonctionnel
e examen *m* funcional
i esame *m* funzionale
n functie-onderzoek *n*
d Funktionsprüfung *f*

1686 PHYSICAL EXAMINATION ROOM
f salle *f* d'examens fonctionnels
e sala *f* de exámenes funcionales
i sala *f* d'esami funzionali
n ruimte voor functie-onderzoeken
d Raum *m* für Funktionsprüfungen

1687 PHYSICAL HEALTH CARE;
SOMATIC HEALTH CARE
f soins *mpl* sanitaires physiques;
soins *mpl* sanitaires somatiques
e cuidado *m* sanitario físico;
atención *f* sanitaria física;
cuidado *m* sanitario somático;
atención *f* sanitaria somática
i cure *fpl* sanitarie fisiche;
cure *fpl* sanitarie somatiche
n lichamelijke gezondheidszorg;
somatische gezondheidszorg
d körperliche Gesundheitspflege *f*;
somatische Gesundheitspflege *f*

1688 PHYSICAL ILLNESS
see: PHYSICAL DISEASE

1689 PHYSICALLY HANDICAPPED DEPARTMENT
f service *m* (département *m*) pour handicapés physiques
e servicio *m* (departamento *m*) para incapacitados corporales
i servizio *m* per handicappati fisici
n afdeling voor lichamelijk gehandicapten
d Abteilung *f* für Körperbehinderte

1690 PHYSICALLY HANDICAPPED UNIT
f unité *f* pour handicapés physiques
e unidad *f* para incapacitados corporales
i unità *f* per handicappati fisici
n eenheid voor lichamelijk gehandicapten
d Station *f* für Körperbehinderte

1691 PHYSICAL MEDICINE
f médecine *f* physique
e medicina *f* física
i medicina *f* fisica
n fysische geneeskunde
d physische Medizin *f*

1692 PHYSICAL MEDICINE DEPARTMENT
f service *m* (département *m*) de médecine physique
e servicio *m* (departamento *m*) de medicina física
i servizio *m* di medicina fisica
n afdeling fysische geneeskunde
d Abteilung *f* für physische Medizin

1693 PHYSICAL PATIENT;
SOMATIC PATIENT
f malade *m* (patient *m*) physique;
malade *m* (patient *m*) somatique
e paciente *m* (enfermo *m*) físico;
paciente *m* (enfermo *m*) somático
i malato *m* fisico;
malato *m* somatico
n lichamelijk zieke;
somatische patiënt
d körperlicher Patient *m* (Kranker *m*);
somatischer Patient *m* (Kranker *m*)

1694 PHYSICAL REHABILITATION
f réadaptation *f* physique
e revalidación *f* física
i riabilitazione *f* fisica
n fysische revalidatie
d körperliche Rehabilitation *f*

1695 PHYSICAL THERAP(EUT)IST;
PHYSIOTHERAP(EUT)IST
f physiothérapeute *m*
e fisioterapeuta *m*
i fisioterapeuta *m*;
fisioterapista *m*
n fysiotherapeut
d Physiotherapeut *m*

1696 PHYSICAL THERAPY;
PHYSIOTHERAPY
f physiothérapie *f*;
thérapie *f* physique
e fisioterapia *f*;
terapia *f* física
i fisioterapia *f*;
terapia *f* fisica
n fysiotherapie;
fysische therapie
d Physiotherapie *f*;
physikalische Therapie *f*

1697 PHYSICAL THERAPY DEPARTMENT;
PHYSIOTHERAPY DEPARTMENT
f service *m* (département *m*) de physiothérapie
e servicio *m* (departamento *m*) de fisioterapia
i servizio *m* di fisioterapia
n afdeling voor fysische therapie
d Abteilung *f* für Physiotherapie;
physiotherapeutische Abteilung *f*

1698 PHYSICIAN
see: DOCTOR

1699 PHYSICIAN-NURSE RELATION
f relation *f* médecin/infirmière
e relación *f* médico/enfermera
i relazione *f* medico/infermiera
n relatie arts/verplegende
d Verhältnis *n* Arzt/Krankenschwester

1700 PHYSICIAN-PATIENT RELATION
f relation *f* médecin/malade
e relación *f* médico/paciente
i relazione *f* medico/paziente
n relatie arts/patiënt
d Verhältnis *n* Arzt/Patient

1701 PHYSICS LABORATORY
f laboratoire *m* de physique
e laboratorio *m* de física
i laboratorio *m* di fisica
n natuurkundig laboratorium *n*
d physikalisches Laboratorium *n*

1702 PHYSIOLOGICAL CHEMISTRY
f chimie *f* physiologique
e química *f* fisiológica
i chimica *f* fisiologica
n fysiologische chemie
d physiologische Chemie *f*

1703 PHYSIOLOGICAL LABORATORY
f laboratoire *m* physiologique
e laboratorio *m* fisiológico
i laboratorio *m* di fisiologia
n fysiologisch laboratorium *n*
d physiologisches Laboratorium *n*

1704 PHYSIOLOGIST
f physiologiste *m*
e fisiólogo *m*
i fisiologo *m*
n fysioloog
d Physiologe *m*

1705 PHYSIOLOGY
f physiologie *f*
e fisiología *f*
i fisiologia *f*
n fysiologie
d Physiologie *f*

1706 PHYSIOTHERAP(EUT)IST
see: PHYSICAL THERAP(EUT)IST

1707 PHYSIOTHERAPY
see: PHYSICAL THERAPY

1708 PHYSIOTHERAPY DEPARTMENT
see: PHYSICAL THERAPY DEPARTMENT

1709 PLANT PHYSICIAN
see: FACTORY PHYSICIAN

1710 PLASMA BANK
f banque *f* de plasma
e banco *m* de plasma
i banca *f* del plasma
n plasmabank
d Plasmabank *f*

1711 PLASTER BED
f lit *m* de plâtre
e cama *f* enyesada
i letto *m* di gesso
n gipsbed *n*
d Gipsbett *n*

1712 PLASTERING TABLE
f table *f* de plâtrage
e mesa *f* enyesada
i tavola *f* di ingessatura
n gipstafel
d Gipstisch *m*

1713 PLASTER ROOM
f salle *f* de plâtre
e sala *f* del yeso;
sala *f* de yesos
i sala *f* dei gessi
n gipskamer
d Gipsraum *m*;
Gipszimmer *n*

1714 PLASTIC SURGEON
f chirurgien *m* plastique
e cirujano *m* plástico
i chirurgo *m* plastico
n plastisch chirurg
d plastischer Chirurg *m*

1715 PLASTIC SURGERY
f chirurgie *f* plastique
e cirugía *f* plástica
i chirurgia *f* plastica
n plastische chirurgie
d plastische Chirurgie *f*

1716 PLASTIC SURGERY CLINIC
f clinique *f* de chirurgie plastique
e clínica *f* de cirugía plástica
i clinica *f* di chirurgia plastica
n kliniek voor plastische chirurgie
d Klinik *f* für plastische Chirurgie

1717 PLASTIC SURGERY DEPARTMENT
f service *m* (département *m*) de chirurgie plastique
e servicio *m* (departamento *m*) de cirugía plástica
i divisione *f* di chirurgia plastica
n afdeling plastische chirurgie
d Abteilung *f* für plastische Chirurgie

1718 PLASTIC SURGERY HOSPITAL
f hôpital *m* de chirurgie plastique
e hospital *m* de cirugía plástica
i ospedale *m* di chirurgia plastica
n ziekenhuis *n* voor plastische chirurgie
d Krankenhaus *n* für plastische Chirurgie

1719 PLASTIC SURGERY UNIT
f unité *f* de chirurgie plastique
e unidad *f* de cirugía plástica
i unità *f* di chirurgia plastica
n eenheid voor plastische chirurgie
d Station *f* für plastische Chirurgie

1720 PLAY THERAPY
f thérapie *f* par le jeu
e terapia *f* del juego
i terapia *f* per mezzo del giuoco
n speltherapie
d Spieltherapie *f*

1721 PNEUMOLOGY
f pneumologie *f*
e neumología *f*
i pneumologia *f*
n pneumologie
d Lungenheilkunde *f*

1722 PNEUMOSURGERY;
PULMONARY SURGERY
f chirurgie *f* pulmonaire
e cirugía *f* pulmonar
i chirurgia *f* polmonare
n longchirurgie
d Lungenchirurgie *f*

1723 PODIATRIST
see: CHIROPODIST

1724 PODIATRY
see: CHIROPODY

1725 POISON CENTRE (CENTER)
f centre *m* anti-poison
e centro *m* antivenenoso
i centro *m* antiveleni
n gif(t)centrum *n*
d Entgiftungszentrum *n*;
Zentrum *n* für Vergiftete

1726 POLYCLINIC
see: OUTPATIENT CARE INSTITUTION

1727 POLYCLINICAL CONSULTATION
see: AMBULATORY CONSULTATION

1728 POLYCLINICAL DEPARTMENT
see: OUTPATIENT DEPARTMENT

1729 POLYCLINICAL SERVICES
see: AMBULATORY CARE SERVICES

1730 POLYCLINICAL TREATMENT
see: AMBULATORY TREATMENT

1731 POPULATION EXAMINATION
f examen *m* de la population
e examen *m* de la población
i esame *m* della popolazione
n bevolkingsonderzoek *n*
d Bevölkerungsuntersuchung *f*

1732 POST-ANESTHETIC DEPARTMENT;
RECOVERY DEPARTMENT
f service *m* (département *m*) de réveil
e servicio *m* (departamento *m*) de recuperación
i servizio *m* di risveglio
n verkoeverafdeling;
recovery-afdeling
d Aufwachabteilung *f*

1733 POST-ANESTHETIC PATIENT;
POST-OPERATIVE PATIENT;
RECOVERY PATIENT
f malade *m* (patient *m*) post-opératoire
e paciente *m* (enfermo *m*) post-operatorio

i malato *m* appena operato
n post-operatieve patiënt;
verkoeverpatiënt
d Frischoperierter *m*;
postoperativer Patient *m*

1734 POST-ANESTHETIC ROOM;
RECOVERY ROOM
f salle *f* de réveil
e sala *f* de recuperación
i sala *f* di risveglio
n verkoeverkamer;
recoverykamer;
uitslaapruimte
d Aufwachraum *m*

1735 POST-ANESTHETIC UNIT;
RECOVERY UNIT
f unité *f* de réveil
e unidad *f* de recuperación
i unità *f* di risveglio
n verkoevereenheid;
recovery-eenheid
d Aufwachstation *f*

1736 POST-HOSPITAL CARE
see: EXTENDED CARE

1737 POST-MORTEM EXAMINATION
see: AUTOPSY

1738 POST-MORTEM ROOM
see: AUTOPSY ROOM

1739 POST-OPERATIVE CARE
f soins *mpl* post-opératoires
e cuidado *m* post-operatorio;
atención *f* post-operatoria
i cure *fpl* post-operatorie
n post-operatieve zorg
d Frischoperiertenpflege *f*;
postoperative Pflege *f*

1740 POST-OPERATIVE DEPARTMENT
f service *m* (département *m*) post-opératoire
e servicio *m* (departamento *m*) post-operatorio
i servizio *m* post-operatorio
n post-operatieve afdeling
d Frischoperiertenabteilung *f*;
postoperative Abteilung *f*

1741 POST-OPERATIVE INTENSIVE CARE
f soins *mpl* post-opératoires intensifs
e cuidado *m* post-operatorio intensivo;
atención *f* post-operatoria intensiva
i cure *fpl* post-operatorie intensive
n post-operatieve intensieve zorg
d Intensivpflege *f* Frischoperierter;
postoperative Intensivpflege *f*

1742 POST-OPERATIVE INTENSIVE CARE DEPARTMENT
f service *m* (département *m*) des soins post-opératoires intensifs
e servicio *m* (departamento *m*) de cuidado post-operatorio intensivo
i servizio *m* di cure post-operatorie intensive
n afdeling voor post-operatieve intensieve zorg
d Intensivpflegeabteilung *f* für Frischoperierte;
postoperative Intensivpflegeabteilung *f*

1743 POST-OPERATIVE PATIENT
see: POST-ANESTHETIC PATIENT

1744 POST-OPERATIVE STAY
f séjour *m* post-opératoire
e estancia *f* post-operatoria
i soggiorno *m* post-operatorio
n post-operatief verblijf *n*
d postoperativer Aufenthalt *m*

1745 POST-OPERATIVE TREATMENT
f traitement *m* post-opératoire
e tratamiento *m* post-operatorio
i trattamento *m* post-operatorio
n post-operatieve behandeling
d Frischoperiertenbehandlung *f*;
postoperative Behandlung *f*

1746 POST-OPERATIVE UNIT
f unité *f* post-opératoire
e unidad *f* post-operatorio
i unità *f* post-operatoria
n post-operatieve eenheid
d Frischoperiertenstation *f*;
postoperative Station *f*

1747 PRACTISING PHYSICIAN;
PRACTITIONER
f praticien *m*
e médico *m* practicante
i medico *m* libero professionista
n praktiserend arts
d niedergelassener Arzt *m*

1748 PRACTITIONER
see: PRACTISING PHYSICIAN

1749 PRE-ADMISSION SCREENING
f examen *m* préliminaire lors de l'admission
e examen *m* preliminar a la admisión
i visita *f* preliminare al momento dell'accettazione
n vooronderzoek *n* bij opname
d Untersuchung *f* vor der Aufnahme

1750 PREGNANCY
f grossesse *f*;
gestation *f*;
gravidité *f*
e embarazo *m*;
preñez *f*;
gravidez *f*
i gravidanza *f*
n zwangerschap
d Schwangerschaft *f*

1751 PRELIMINARY NURSES' SCHOOL
see: NURSES' PREPARATORY TRAINING SCHOOL

1752 PRELIMINARY NURSE TRAINING SCHOOL
see: NURSES' PREPARATORY TRAINING SCHOOL

1753 PRELIMINARY NURSING SCHOOL
see: NURSES' PREPARATORY TRAINING SCHOOL

1754 PREMATURE BABY CARE;
PREMATURE INFANT CARE
f soins *mpl* aux prématurés
e cuidado *m* (atención *f*) de los prematuros
i cura *f* dei neonati immaturi
n verzorging van prematuren
d Frühgeborenenpflege *f*

1755 PREMATURE BABY DEPARTMENT;
PREMATURE INFANT DEPARTMENT
f service *m* (département *m*) pour prématurés

e servicio *m* (departamento *m*) para prematuros
i reparto *m* dei neonati immaturi
n prematurenafdeling
d Frühgeborenenabteilung *f*

1756 PREMATURE DISCHARGE
f décharge *f* anticipée;
démission *f* anticipée;
sortie *f* anticipée;
licenciement *m* anticipé
e egreso *m* anticipado;
salida *f* anticipada;
alta *f* anticipada;
despido *m* anticipado
i dimissione *f* anticipata;
uscita *f* anticipata
n vervroegd ontslag *n*
d verfrühte Entlassung *f*

1757 PREMATURE INFANT CARE
see: PREMATURE BABY CARE

1758 PREMATURE INFANT DEPARTMENT
see: PREMATURE BABY DEPARTMENT

1759 PRENATAL CLINIC
f clinique *f* prénatale
e clínica *f* prenatal
i clinica *f* prenatale
n prenatale kliniek
d pränatale Klinik *f*

1760 PRENATAL CONSULTATION
f consultation *f* prénatale
e consulta *f* prenatal
i consulto *m* prenatale
n prenatale consultatie
d Schwangerenberatung *f*

1761 PRE-NURSING SCHOOL
see: NURSES' PREPARATORY TRAINING SCHOOL

1762 PRE-OPERATIVE CARE
f soins *mpl* pré-opératoires
e cuidado *m* pre-operatorio;
atención *f* pre-operatoria
i cure *fpl* pre-operatorie
n pre-operatieve zorg
d präoperative Pflege *f*

1763 PRE-OPERATIVE PATIENT
f malade *m* (patient *m*) pré-opératoire
e paciente *m* (enfermo *m*) pre-operatorio
i malato *m* pre-operatorio
n pre-operatieve patiënt
d präoperativer Patient *m*

1764 PRE-OPERATIVE ROOM;
PREPARATIONS ROOM
f salle *f* préparatoire;
salle *f* de préparation
e sala *f* preparatoria
i sala *f* di preparazione
n voorbereidingskamer
d Vorbereitungsraum *m*

1765 PRE-OPERATIVE STAY
f séjour *m* pré-opératoire
e estancia *f* pre-operatoria
i soggiorno *m* pre-operatorio
n pre-operatief verblijf *n*
d präoperativer Aufenthalt *m*

1766 PRE-OPERATIVE TREATMENT
f traitement *m* pré-opératoire
e tratamiento *m* pre-operatorio
i trattamento *m* pre-operatorio
n pre-operatieve behandeling
d präoperative Behandlung *f*

1767 PREPARATIONS ROOM
see: PRE-OPERATIVE ROOM

1768 PREVENTIVE HEALTH CARE
f soins *mpl* sanitaires préventifs
e cuidado *m* sanitario preventivo;
atención *f* sanitaria preventiva
i cure *fpl* sanitarie preventive
n preventieve gezondheidszorg
d präventive Gesundheitsfürsorge *f*;
präventive Gesundheitspflege *f*;
Gesundheitsvorsorge *f*

1769 PREVENTIVE HEALTH SERVICES
f services *mpl* sanitaires préventifs
e servicios *mpl* sanitarios preventivos;
servicios *mpl* de salud preventivos
i servizi *mpl* sanitari preventivi
n preventieve gezondheidsdiensten
d präventive Gesundheitsfürsorgedienste *mpl*

1770 PREVENTIVE MEDICINE
f médecine *f* préventive
e medicina *f* preventiva
i medicina *f* preventiva
n preventieve geneeskunde
d präventive Medizin *f*;
Präventivmedizin *f*;
Vorsorgemedizin *f*

1771 PREVENTIVE MENTAL HEALTH CARE
f soins *mpl* mentaux préventifs
e cuidado *m* mental preventivo;
atención *f* mental preventiva
i cure *fpl* mentali preventive
n preventieve geestelijke gezondheidszorg
d präventive psychiatrische Fürsorge *f*

1772 PREVENTIVE MENTAL HEALTH SERVICES
f services *mpl* de soins mentaux préventifs
e servicios *mpl* de cuidado mental preventivo
i servizi *mpl* di cure mentali preventive
n voorzieningen voor preventieve geestelijke gezondheidszorg
d Dienste *mpl* für präventive psychiatrische Fürsorge

1773 PREVENTIVE PEDIATRICS
f pédiatrie *f* préventive
e pediatría *f* preventiva
i pediatria *f* preventiva
n preventieve pediatrie
d präventive Pädiatrie *f*

1774 PRICE AGREEMENT
f contrat *m* tarifaire
e contrato *m* de tarifas
i contratto *m* tariffario
n tariefovereenkomst
d Tarifvertrag *m*

1775 PRIMARY CARE
see: BASIC CARE

1776 PRISON HOSPITAL
f hôpital *m* de prison

e hospital *m* de prisión
i ospedale *m* di prigione
n gevangenisziekenhuis *n*
d Gefängniskrankenhaus *n*

1777 PRIVATE BED
f lit *m* privé
e cama *f* privada
i letto *m* privato;
letto *m* a pagamento
n bed *n* voor particuliere patiënten
d Privatbett *n*

1778 PRIVATE CLINIC
f clinique *f* privée
e clínica *f* privada
i clinica *f* privata
n privé-kliniek
d Privatklinik *f*

1779 PRIVATE FEE
f honoraires *mpl* privés
e honorarios *mpl* privados
i onorari *mpl* privati
n particulier honorarium *n*
d Privathonorar *n*

1780 PRIVATE HEALTH CARE INSTITUTION;
PRIVATE HEALTH INSTITUTION
f établissement *m* sanitaire privé;
établissement *m* de santé privé;
institution *f* sanitaire privée;
institution *f* de santé privée
e institución *f* sanitaria privada;
institución *f* de salud privada;
instalación *f* sanitaria privada;
instalación *f* de salud privada
i istituto *m* sanitario privato;
stabilimento *m* sanitario privato
n particuliere instelling (inrichting) voor gezondheidszorg
d private Gesundheits(pflege)einrichtung *f*

1781 PRIVATE HEALTH INSTITUTION
see: PRIVATE HEALTH CARE INSTITUTION

1782 PRIVATE HEALTH INSURANCE
f assurance-maladie *f* privée
e seguro *m* de enfermedad privado;
seguro *m* de salud privado
i assicurazione *f* malattia privata;
assicurazione *f* privata contro le malattie
n particuliere ziekte(kosten)verzekering
d private Krankenversicherung *f*

1783 PRIVATE HEALTH INSURANCE COMPANY
f compagnie *f* d'assurance-maladie privée
e compañía *f* de seguro de enfermedad privado
i compagnia *f* di assicurazione malattia privata
n particuliere ziekte(kosten)verzekeraar;
particuliere ziekte(kosten)verzekeringsmaatschappij
d private Krankenversicherungsgesellschaft *f*

1784 PRIVATE HOSPITAL
f hôpital *m* privé;
établissement *m* hospitalier privé;
établissement *m* d'hospitalisation privé;
institution *f* hospitalière privée
e hospital *m* privado;
institución *f* hospitalaria privada
i ospedale *m* privato;
stabilimento *m* ospedaliero privato
n privé-ziekenhuis *n*;
particulier ziekenhuis *n*
d privates Krankenhaus *n*;
Privatkrankenhaus *n*;
private Krankenanstalt *f*;
Privatkrankenanstalt *f*;
nicht-öffentliches Krankenhaus *n*

1785 PRIVATE HOSPITALIZATION
f hospitalisation *f* privée
e hospitalización *f* privada
i ospedalizzazione *f* privata;
ospedalizzazione *f* a pagamento
n opneming in een privé-ziekenhuis;
opneming in een particulier ziekenhuis
d Einweisung *f* in ein Privatkrankenhaus

1786 PRIVATE MEDICINE
f médecine *f* privée;
médecine *f* de clientèle
e medicina *f* privada
i medicina *f* privata;
medicina *f* clientelare
n particuliere geneeskunde
d Privatmedizin *f*

1787 PRIVATE NON-PROFIT HOSPITAL;
PRIVATE NON-PROFIT MAKING HOSPITAL
f hôpital *m* privé sans but lucratif;
établissement *m* hospitalier privé sans but lucratif
e hospital *m* privado sin fines de lucro
i ospedale *m* privato senza fine lucrativo
n particulier ziekenhuis *n* zonder winstoogmerk;
particulier non-profit ziekenhuis *n*
d privat-gemeinnütziges Krankenhaus *n*

1788 PRIVATE NON-PROFIT MAKING HOSPITAL
see: PRIVATE NON-PROFIT HOSPITAL

1789 PRIVATE PATIENT
f malade *m* (patient *m*) privé;
malade *m* (patient *m*) payant
e paciente *m* (enfermo *m*) de pago
i malato *m* (paziente *m*) pagante
n particuliere patiënt;
klassepatiënt
d Privatpatient *m*;
Privatkranker *m*

1790 PRIVATE PATIENTS DEPARTMENT
f service *m* (département *m*) pour malades privés
e servicio *m* (departamento *m*) para pacientes de pago
i servizio *m* per malati paganti
n klasse(kamer)afdeling
d Privatabteilung *f*

1791 PRIVATE PHYSICIAN
f médecin *m* privé
e médico *m* privado
i medico *m* privato;
medico *m* professionista;
medico *m* che esercita la libera professione
n arts met particuliere praktijk
d Privatarzt *m*

1792 PRIVATE PRACTICE
f pratique *f* privée
e práctica *f* privada
i pratica *f* privata
n particuliere praktijk
d Privatpraxis *f*

1793 PRIVATE PROFIT HOSPITAL;
PRIVATE PROFIT MAKING HOSPITAL
f hôpital *m* privé à but lucratif;
établissement *m* hospitalier privé à but lucratif
e hospital *m* privado con fines de lucro
i ospedale *m* privato a fine lucrativo
n particulier ziekenhuis *n* met winstoogmerk;
particulier profit-ziekenhuis *n*
d privat-gewerbliches Krankenhaus *n*

1794 PRIVATE PROFIT MAKING HOSPITAL
see: PRIVATE PROFIT HOSPITAL

1795 PRIVATE ROOM
f chambre *f* privée
e cuarto *m* particular
i camera *f* a pagamento
n klassekamer
d Privatzimmer *n*

1796 PROFESSIONAL LIABILITY
f responsabilité *f* professionnelle
e responsabilidad *f* profesional
i responsabilità *f* professionale
n beroepsverantwoordelijkheid;
beroepsaansprakelijkheid
d Berufshaftpflicht *f*

1797 PROFESSIONAL REHABILITATION;
VOCATIONAL REHABILITATION
f réadaptation *f* professionnelle
e revalidación *f* profesional
i riabilitazione *f* professionale
n beroepsrevalidatie
d berufliche Rehabilitation *f*

1798 PROFESSIONAL SECRET
f secret *m* professionnel
e secreto *m* profesional;
sigilo *m* profesional
i segreto *m* professionale
n beroepsgeheim *n*
d Berufsgeheimnis *n*

1799 PROFIT HOSPITAL;
PROFIT MAKING HOSPITAL
f hôpital *m* à but lucratif;
établissement *m* hospitalier à but lucratif
e hospital *m* con fines de lucro
i ospedale *m* a fine lucrativo
n ziekenhuis *n* met winstoogmerk;
profit-ziekenhuis *n*
d gewerbliches Krankenhaus *n*

1800 PROFIT MAKING HOSPITAL
see: PROFIT HOSPITAL

1801 PROGRESSIVE CARE
f soins *mpl* progressifs
e cuidado *m* progresivo;
atención *f* progresiva
i cure *fpl* progressive
n progressieve zorg
d Progressivpflege *f*;
progressive Pflege *f*;
fortschrittliche Pflege *f*

1802 PROGRESSIVE TREATMENT
f traitement *m* progressif
e tratamiento *m* progresivo
i trattamento *m* progressivo
n progressieve behandeling
d Progressivbehandlung *f*;
progressive Behandlung *f*;
fortschrittliche Behandlung *f*

1803 PROPHYLAXIS
f prophylaxie *f*
e profilaxia *f*;
profilaxis *f*
i profilassi *f*
n profylaxe
d Prophylaxe *f*

1804 PROSTHESIS
f prothèse *f*
e prótesis *f*
i protesi *f*
n prothese
d Prothese *f*

1805 PROSTHETIC TECHNICIAN
f mécanicien *m* spécialisé en prothèses orthopédiques
e mecánico *m* ortopédico
i meccanico *m* specializzato in protesi ortepediche
n orthopedisch instrumentmaker
d Orthopädiemechaniker *m*

1806 PROTECTED EMPLOYMENT;
PROTECTED WORK;
SHELTERED EMPLOYMENT;
SHELTERED WORK
f travail *m* protégé;
emploi *m* protégé;
travail *m* réservé;
emploi *m* réservé
e trabajo *m* protegido;
ocupación *f* protegida;
trabajo *m* a cubierto;
ocupación *f* a cubierto
i lavoro *m* protetto;
impiego *m* protetto;
lavoro *m* riservato agli handicappati mentali;
impiego *m* riservato agli handicappati mentali
n beschutte arbeid;
beschutte tewerkstelling;
beschut werk *n*
d geschützte Beschäftigung *f*;
wettbewerbsgeschützte Beschäftigung *f*

1807 PROTECTED WORK
see: PROTECTED EMPLOYMENT

1808 PROTECTED WORKSHOP;
SHELTERED WORKSHOP
f atelier *m* protégé;
établissement *m* de travail protégé
e taller *m* protegido;
taller *m* abrigado;
taller *m* al abrigo;
taller *m* social
i luogo *m* di lavoro protetto;
luogo *m* di lavoro riservato agli handicappati mentali
n beschutte werkplaats;
sociale werkplaats;
beschermde werkplaats
d geschützte Werkstatt *f*;
geschützte Werkstätte *f*;
wettbewerbsgeschützte Werkstatt *f*;
wettbewerbsgeschützte Werkstätte *f*

1809 PSYCHIATRIC BED
f lit *m* psychiatrique;
lit *m* de psychiatrie

e cama *f* psiquiátrica;
cama *f* de psiquiatría
i letto *m* psichiatrico
n psychiatrisch bed *n*
d psychiatrisches Bett *n*;
Bett *n* für psychiatrische Fälle

1810 PSYCHIATRIC CARE
see: MENTAL CARE

1811 PSYCHIATRIC CENTRE (CENTER)
see: MENTAL HEALTH CENTRE (CENTER)

1812 PSYCHIATRIC CLINIC
see: MENTAL HEALTH CLINIC

1813 PSYCHIATRIC DAY HOSPITAL
f hôpital *m* psychiatrique de jour
e hospital *m* psiquiátrico diurno
i ospedale *m* psichiatrico diurno
n psychiatrisch dagziekenhuis *n*
d psychiatrisches Tageskrankenhaus *n*

1814 PSYCHIATRIC DEPARTMENT
see: MENTAL DISEASES DEPARTMENT

1815 PSYCHIATRIC DEPARTMENT IN A GENERAL HOSPITAL
see: MENTAL DISEASES DEPARTMENT IN A GENERAL HOSPITAL

1816 PSYCHIATRIC DISEASE
see: MENTAL DISEASE

1817 PSYCHIATRIC EMERGENCY SERVICES
f services *mpl* psychiatriques d'urgence
e servicios *mpl* psiquiátricos de urgencia
i servizi *mpl* psichiatrici d'urgenza
n psychiatrische diensten voor spoedgevallen
d psychiatrische Notfalldienste *mpl*

1818 PSYCHIATRIC FACILITIES
see: MENTAL HEALTH FACILITIES

1819 PSYCHIATRIC HOME CARE
f soins *mpl* psychiatriques à domicile
e cuidado *m* psiquiátrico domiciliario;
atención *f* psiquiátrica domiciliaria
i cure *fpl* psichiatriche domiciliari
n psychiatrische thuisverzorging
d psychiatrische Heimversorgung *f*

1820 PSYCHIATRIC HOSPITAL
see: MENTAL DISEASES HOSPITAL

1821 PSYCHIATRIC ILLNESS
see: MENTAL DISEASE

1822 PSYCHIATRIC INSTITUTION
see: MENTAL DISEASES HOSPITAL

1823 PSYCHIATRIC NURSE
f infirmière *f* psychiatrique
e enfermera *f* psiquiátrica;
enfermera *f* psiquiatra
i infermiera *f* psichiatrica
n psychiatrisch verpleegkundige;
psychiatrische verplegende;
B-verplegende
d Psychiatriepflegerin *f*;
Psychiatrieschwester *f*

1824 PSYCHIATRIC NURSING
f soins *mpl* infirmiers psychiatriques
e enfermería *f* psiquiátrica
i cure *fpl* infermieristiche psichiatriche
n psychiatrische verpleging
d psychiatrische Krankenpflege *f*;
geistige Krankenpflege *f*

1825 PSYCHIATRIC NURSING DEPARTMENT
f service *m* (département *m*) de soins psychiatriques
e servicio *m* (departamento *m*) de cuidado psiquiátrico
i servizio *m* di cure psichiatriche
n psychiatrische verpleegafdeling
d psychiatrische Pflegeabteilung *f*

1826 PSYCHIATRIC NURSING UNIT
f unité *f* de soins psychiatriques
e unidad *f* de cuidado psiquiátrico
i unità *f* di cure psichiatriche
n psychiatrische verpleegeenheid
d psychiatrische Pflegestation *f*

1827 PSYCHIATRIC OUTPATIENT DEPARTMENT
f service *m* (département *m*) de consultations psychiatriques externes
e servicio *m* (departamento *m*) de consultas psiquiátricas externas
i ambulatorio *m* psichiatrico esterno
n psychiatrische polikliniek
d psychiatrische Poliklinik *f*

1828 PSYCHIATRIC PATIENT
see: MENTAL PATIENT

1829 PSYCHIATRIC RESEARCH
f recherche *f* psychiatrique
e investigación *f* psiquiátrica
i ricerca *f* psichiatrica
n psychiatrisch onderzoekswerk *n*;
psychiatrische research
d psychiatrische Forschung *f*

1830 PSYCHIATRIC SERVICES
see: MENTAL HEALTH FACILITIES

1831 PSYCHIATRIC SOCIAL WORK
f assistance *f* sociale psychiatrique
e asistencia *f* social psiquiátrica
i assistenza *f* sociale psichiatrica
n psychiatrisch sociaal werk *n*
d psychiatrische Sozialhilfe *f*

1832 PSYCHIATRIC SOCIAL WORKER
f assistant *m* social psychiatrique
e asistente *m* social psiquiátrico
i assistente *m* sociale di psichiatria
n psychiatrisch maatschappelijk werker;
psychiatrisch sociaal werker
d psychiatrischer Sozialfürsorger *m*;
psychiatrischer Sozialarbeiter *m*

1833 PSYCHIATRIC STUDENT NURSE
f élève-infirmière *f* psychiatrique
e enfermera *f* alumna psiquiátrica
i allieva *f* infermiera psichiatrica
n psychiatrische leerling-verpleegkundige;
leerling B-verpleegkunde
d psychiatrische Pflegeschülerin *f*

1834 PSYCHIATRIC TEACHING HOSPITAL
f hôpital *m* d'enseignement psychiatrique
e hospital *m* docente psiquiátrico

i ospedale *m* d'insegnamento psichiatrico
n psychiatrisch opleidingsziekenhuis *n*
d psychiatrisches Ausbildungskrankenhaus *n*

1835 PSYCHIATRIC TREATMENT
f traitement *m* psychiatrique
e tratamiento *m* psiquiátrico
i trattamento *m* psichiatrico
n psychiatrische behandeling
d psychiatrische Behandlung *f*

1836 PSYCHIATRIC UNIT
see: MENTAL DISEASES UNIT

1837 PSYCHIATRIC UNIT IN A GENERAL HOSPITAL
see: MENTAL DISEASES UNIT IN A GENERAL HOSPITAL

1838 PSYCHIATRIST
f psychiatre *m*
e psiquiatra *m*
i psichiatra *m*
n psychiater
d Psychiater *m*

1839 PSYCHIATRY
f psychiatrie *f*
e psiquiatría *f*
i psichiatria *f*
n psychiatrie
d Psychiatrie *f*

1840 PSYCHIATRY DEPARTMENT
see: MENTAL DISEASES DEPARTMENT

1841 PSYCHIATRY DEPARTMENT IN A GENERAL HOSPITAL
see: MENTAL DISEASES DEPARTMENT IN A GENERAL HOSPITAL

1842 PSYCHIATRY FACILITIES
see: MENTAL HEALTH FACILITIES

1843 PSYCHIATRY HOSPITAL
see: MENTAL DISEASES HOSPITAL

1844 PSYCHIATRY SERVICES
see: MENTAL HEALTH FACILITIES

1845 PSYCHIATRY UNIT
see: MENTAL DISEASES UNIT

1846 PSYCHIATRY UNIT IN A GENERAL HOSPITAL
see: MENTAL DISEASES UNIT IN A GENERAL HOSPITAL

1847 PSYCHOGERIATRIC DEPARTMENT
f service *m* (département *m*) psychogériatrique;
service *m* (département *m*) de psychogériatrie
e servicio *m* (departamento *m*) psicogeriátrico;
servicio *m* (departamento *m*) de psicogeriatría
i divisione *f* di geronto-psichiatria
n psychogeriatrische afdeling;
gerontopsychiatrische afdeling
d psychogeriatrische Abteilung *f*

1848 PSYCHOGERIATRIC HOSPITAL
f hôpital *m* psychogériatrique;
hôpital *m* de psychogériatrie
e hospital *m* psicogeriátrico;
hospital *m* de psicogeriatría
i ospedale *m* geronto-psichiatrico
n psychogeriatrisch ziekenhuis *n*;
gerontopsychiatrisch ziekenhuis *n*
d psychogeriatrisches Krankenhaus *n*

1849 PSYCHOGERIATRIC PATIENT
f malade *m* (patient *m*) psychogériatrique
e paciente *m* (enfermo *m*) psicogeriátrico
i malato *m* geronto-psichiatrico
n psychisch gestoorde bejaarde;
psychogeriatrische patiënt;
gerontopsychiatrische patiënt
d psychogeriatrischer Patient *m*

1850 PSYCHOGERIATRICS
f psychogériatrie *f*
e psicogeriatría *f*
i geronto-psichiatria *f*
n psychogeriatrie;
gerontopsychiatrie
d Psychogeriatrie *f*

1851 PSYCHOGERIATRIC SERVICES
f services *mpl* psychogériatriques;
services *mpl* de psychogériatrie
e servicios *mpl* psicogeriátricos;
servicios *mpl* de psicogeriatría
i servizi *mpl* di geronto-psichiatria
n psychogeriatrische diensten;
gerontopsychiatrische diensten
d psychogeriatrische Dienste *mpl*

1852 PSYCHOGERIATRIC UNIT
f unité *f* psychogériatrique;
unité *f* de psychogériatrie
e unidad *f* psicogeriátrica;
unidad *f* de psicogeriatría
i unità *f* di geronto-psichiatria
n psychogeriatrische eenheid;
gerontopsychiatrische eenheid
d psychogeriatrische Station *f*

1853 PSYCHOLOGIST
f psychologue *m*
e psicólogo *m*
i psicologo *m*
n psycholoog
d Psychologe *m*

1854 PSYCHOLOGY
f psychologie *f*
e psicología *f*
i psicologia *f*
n psychologie
d Psychologie *f*

1855 PSYCHOSOMATIC MEDICINE
f médecine *f* psychosomatique
e medicina *f* psicosomática
i medicina *f* psicosomatica
n psychosomatische geneeskunde
d psychosomatische Medizin *f*

1856 PSYCHOTECHNICIAN
f psychotechnicien *m*
e psicotécnico *m*
i psicotecnico *m*
n psychotechnicus
d Psychotechniker *m*

1857 PSYCHOTHERAPEUTIC CENTRE (CENTER)
PSYCHOTHERAPY CENTRE (CENTER)
f centre *m* psychothérapeutique

e centro *m* psicoterapéutico
i centro *m* psicoterapico
n psychotherapeutisch centrum *n*
d psychotherapeutisches Zentrum *n*

1858 PSYCHOTHERAPY
f psychothérapie *f*
e psicoterapia *f*
i psicoterapia *f*
n psychotherapie
d Psychotherapie *f*

1859 PSYCHOTHERAPY CENTRE (CENTER)
see: PSYCHOTHERAPEUTIC CENTRE (CENTER)

1860 PUBLIC HEALTH
f santé *f* publique
e salud *f* pública;
sanidad *f* pública
i sanità *f* pubblica
n volksgezondheid
d Volksgesundheit *f*;
Gesundheitswesen *n*;
öffentliche Gesundheit *f*

1861 PUBLIC HEALTH AUTHORITIES
f autorités *fpl* de santé publique
e autoridades *fpl* de salud pública
i autorità *fpl* di sanità pubblica
n overheden voor de volksgezondheid
d Behörden *fpl* der öffentlichen Gesundheitsfürsorge

1862 PUBLIC HEALTH BUDGET
f budget *m* de santé publique
e presupuesto *m* de salud pública
i budget *m* di sanità pubblica
n budget *n* voor volksgezondheid
d öffentliches Gesundheitsbudget *n*

1863 PUBLIC HEALTH CARE
f soins *mpl* sanitaires publics;
soins *mpl* de santé publique
e cuidado *m* sanitario público;
atención *f* sanitaria pública
i assistenza *f* sanitaria pubblica
n openbare gezondheidszorg
d öffentliche Gesundheitsfürsorge *f*;
öffentliche Gesundheitspflege *f*

1864 PUBLIC HEALTH CARE INSTITUTION;
PUBLIC HEALTH INSTITUTION
f établissement *m* de santé publique;
institution *f* de santé publique
e institución *f* de salud pública;
instalación *f* de salud pública
i istituto *m* sanitario pubblico;
stabilimento *m* sanitario pubblico
n instelling voor openbare gezondheidszorg;
inrichting voor openbare gezondheidszorg
d Einrichtung *f* der öffentlichen Gesundheit(spflege);
Einrichtung *f* des öffentlichen Gesundheitswesens

1865 PUBLIC HEALTH CARE INSURANCE;
PUBLIC HEALTH (COSTS) INSURANCE
f assurance-maladie *f* publique;
assurance *f* publique contre la maladie
e seguro *m* de enfermedad público;
seguro *m* de salud público
i assicurazione *f* pubblica contro le malattie
n volksverzekering tegen ziektekosten
d öffentliche Krankenversicherung *f*

1866 PUBLIC HEALTH CARE MANAGEMENT;
PUBLIC HEALTH MANAGEMENT
f gestion *f* de la santé publique
e gestión *f* de salud pública
i gestione *f* della sanità pubblica
n beleid *n* inzake volksgezondheid
d Verwaltung *f* der öffentlichen Gesundheitsfürsorge

1867 PUBLIC HEALTH CARE POLICY;
PUBLIC HEALTH POLICY
f politique *f* de la santé publique
e política *f* de salud pública
i politica *f* della sanità pubblica
n volksgezondheidspolitiek
d Politik *f* der öffentlichen Gesundheitsfürsorge

1868 PUBLIC HEALTH CARE SERVICES;
PUBLIC HEALTH SERVICES
f services *mpl* sanitaires publics;
services *mpl* de santé publique
e servicios *mpl* sanitarios públicos;
servicios *mpl* de salud pública;
servicios *mpl* de sanidad pública
i servizi *mpl* sanitari pubblici
n volksgezondheidsdiensten
d Dienste *mpl* für öffentliche Gesundheitsfürsorge

1869 PUBLIC HEALTH CARE SYSTEM;
PUBLIC HEALTH SYSTEM
f système *m* sanitaire public;
système *m* de la santé publique
e sistema *m* sanitario público;
sistema *m* de salud pública
i organizzazione *f* della sanità pubblica
n systeem *n* van de openbare gezondheidszorg
d System *n* des öffentlichen Gesundheitswesens

1870 PUBLIC HEALTH COSTS INSURANCE
see: PUBLIC HEALTH CARE INSURANCE

1871 PUBLIC HEALTH INSTITUTION
see: PUBLIC HEALTH CARE INSTITUTION

1872 PUBLIC HEALTH INSURANCE
see: PUBLIC HEALTH CARE INSURANCE

1873 PUBLIC HEALTH MANAGEMENT
see: PUBLIC HEALTH CARE MANAGEMENT

1874 PUBLIC HEALTH POLICY
see: PUBLIC HEALTH CARE POLICY

1875 PUBLIC HEALTH SCHOOL
f école *f* de la santé publique
e escuela *f* de salud pública
i scuola *f* di sanità pubblica
n school voor openbare gezondheidszorg
d Schule *f* des Gesundheitswesens

1876 PUBLIC HEALTH SERVICES
see: PUBLIC HEALTH CARE SERVICES

1877 PUBLIC HEALTH SYSTEM
see: PUBLIC HEALTH CARE SYSTEM

1878 PUBLIC HOSPITAL
f hôpital *m* public;
établissement *m* hospitalier public;
établissement *m* public d'hospitalisation;
institution *f* hospitalière publique

e hospital *m* público;
hospital *m* oficial;
institución *f* hospitalaria pública
i ospedale *m* pubblico;
stabilimento *m* ospedaliero pubblico
n openbaar ziekenhuis *n*;
overheidsziekenhuis *n*
d öffentliches Krankenhaus *n*;
öffentlich-rechtliches Krankenhaus *n*;
frei-gemeinnütziges Krankenhaus *n*

1879 PUBLIC HOSPITALIZATION
f hospitalisation *f* publique
e hospitalización *f* pública
i ospedalizzazione *f* pubblica
n opneming in een openbaar ziekenhuis
d Einweisung *f* in ein öffentliches Krankenhaus

1880 PULMONARY CLINIC
f clinique *f* pulmonaire
e clínica *f* pulmonar
i clinica *f* delle malattie polmonari;
clinica *f* pneumologica
n longkliniek
d Lungenklinik *f*

1881 PULMONARY DEPARTMENT
f service *m* (département *m*) pulmonaire
e servicio *m* (departamento *m*) pulmonar
i divisione *f* delle malattie polmonari;
divisione *f* pneumologica
n longafdeling
d Lungenabteilung *f*

1882 PULMONARY DISEASE
f maladie *f* pulmonaire;
péripneumonie *f*
e enfermedad *f* pulmonar
i malattia *f* polmonare
n longziekte
d Lungenkrankheit *f*

1883 PULMONARY HOSPITAL
f hôpital *m* pulmonaire
e hospital *m* pulmonar
i ospedale *m* per malattie polmonari;
ospedale *m* pneumologico
n longziekenhuis *n*
d Lungenkrankenhaus *n*

1884 PULMONARY SURGERY
see: PNEUMOSURGERY

1885 PULMONARY UNIT
f unité *f* pulmonaire
e unidad *f* pulmonar
i unità *f* delle malattie polmonari;
unità *f* pneumologica
n longeenheid
d Lungenstation *f*

1886 PUPIL MIDWIFE;
PUPIL OBSTETRICIAN
f élève-accoucheuse *f*
e partera *f* alumna;
comadre *f* alumna;
matrona *f* alumna
i allieva *f* levatrice;
allieva *f* ostetrica
n leerling-vroedvrouw;
leerling-verloskundige
d Hebammeschülerin *f*

1887 PUPIL NURSE
see: NURSING STUDENT

1888 PUPIL OBSTETRICIAN
see: PUPIL MIDWIFE

R

1889 RADIATION HAZARD
f danger *m* de radiation
e peligro *m* de radiación
i pericolo *m* di radiazioni
n stralingsgevaar *n*
d Strahlungsgefahr *f*

1890 RADIATION PROTECTION
f protection *f* contre les radiations
e protección *f* contra radiaciones
i protezione *f* contro le radiazioni
n stralingsbescherming
d Strahlenschutz *m*

1891 RADIOCHEMICAL LABORATORY
f laboratoire *m* radiochimique;
laboratoire *m* de radiochimie
e laboratorio *m* radioquímico;
laboratorio *m* de radioquímica
i laboratorio *m* radiochimico;
laboratorio *m* di radiochimica
n radiochemisch laboratorium *n*
d radiochemisches Laboratorium *n*

1892 RADIODIAGNOSTICS
f radiodiagnostic *m*
e radiodiagnóstico *m*
i radiodiagnostica *f*
n röntgendiagnostiek
d Röntgendiagnostik *f*

1893 RADIOGRAPH;
X-RAY PICTURE
f radiographie *f*
e radiografía *f*;
roentgenografía *f*
i radiografia *f*
n röntgenfoto
d Röntgenaufnahme *f*

1894 RADIOGRAPHY;
X-RAY EXAMINATION
f examen *m* radiographique
e examen *m* radiológico;
examen *m* mediante (por) rayos x
i esame *m* radiologico;
esame *m* radioscopico
n röntgenonderzoek *n*
d Röntgenuntersuchung *f*

1895 RADIOGRAPHY ROOM
f salle *f* de radiographie
e sala *f* de radiografía
i sala *f* di radiografia
n radiografieruimte
d Röntgensaal *m*

1896 RADIOISOTOPES DEPARTMENT
f service *m* (département *m*) de radio-isotopes;
service *m* (département *m*) d'isotopes radio-actifs
e servicio *m* (departamento *m*) de radioisótopos
i servizio *m* isotopi radioattivi
n isotopenafdeling
d Isotopenabteilung *f*

1897 RADIOLOGICAL APPARATUS;
RADIOLOGY APPARATUS;
X-RAY APPARATUS
f appareils *mpl* radiologiques;
appareils *mpl* de rayons x
e aparatos *mpl* radiológicos;
aparatos *mpl* de rayos x
i apparecchi *mpl* radiologici
n röntgenapparatuur
d Röntgengeräte *npl*

1898 RADIOLOGICAL DEPARTMENT;
RADIOLOGY DEPARTMENT;
X-RAY DEPARTMENT
f service *m* (département *m*) radiologique;
service *m* (département *m*) de radiologie;
service *m* (département *m*) de rayons x
e servicio *m* (departamento *m*) radiológico;
servicio *m* (departamento *m*) de radiología;
servicio *m* (departamento *m*) de rayos x
i servizio *m* di radiologia;
servizio *m* dei raggi x
n röntgenafdeling;
radiologische afdeling;
radiologie-afdeling
d Röntgenabteilung *f*;
radiologische Abteilung *f*;
Radiologieabteilung *f*

1899 RADIOLOGICAL PERSONNEL;
RADIOLOGICAL STAFF;
RADIOLOGY PERSONNEL;
RADIOLOGY STAFF;
X-RAY PERSONNEL;
X-RAY STAFF
f personnel *m* de radiologie
e personal *m* de radiología
i personale *m* di radiologia
n röntgenpersoneel *n*
d Röntgenpersonal *n*

1900 RADIOLOGICAL ROOM;
RADIOLOGY ROOM;
X-RAY ROOM
f salle *f* radiologique;
salle *f* de radiologie;
salle *f* de rayons x
e sala *f* radiológica;
sala *f* de radiología;
sala *f* de rayos x
i sala *f* di radiologia;
sala *f* dei raggi x
n röntgenkamer
d Röntgenraum *m*;
Röntgenzimmer *n*

1901 RADIOLOGICAL STAFF
see: RADIOLOGICAL PERSONNEL

1902 RADIOLOGICAL TECHNOLOGY;
RADIOLOGY TECHNOLOGY;
X-RAY TECHNOLOGY
f technologie *f* radiologique
e tecnología *f* radiológica
i tecnologia *f* radiologica

n röntgentechnologie
d Röntgentechnologie *f*

1903 RADIOLOGICAL UNIT;
RADIOLOGY UNIT;
X-RAY UNIT
f unité *f* radiologique;
unité *f* de radiologie;
unité *f* de rayons x
e unidad *f* radiológica;
unidad *f* de radiología;
unidad *f* de rayos x
i unità *f* di radiologia;
unità *f* dei raggi x
n röntgeneenheid
d Röntgenstation *f*

1904 RADIOLOGIST
f radiologue *m*;
radiologiste *m*
e radiólogo *m*;
roentgenólogo *m*
i radiologo *m*
n radioloog;
röntgenoloog
d Röntgenologe *m*

1905 RADIOLOGY
f radiologie *f*
e radiología *f*
i radiologia *f*
n radiologie
d Radiologie *f*

1906 RADIOLOGY APPARATUS
see: RADIOLOGICAL APPARATUS

1907 RADIOLOGY DEPARTMENT
see: RADIOLOGICAL DEPARTMENT

1908 RADIOLOGY PERSONNEL
see: RADIOLOGICAL PERSONNEL

1909 RADIOLOGY ROOM
see: RADIOLOGICAL ROOM

1910 RADIOLOGY STAFF
see: RADIOLOGICAL PERSONNEL

1911 RADIOLOGY TECHNOLOGY
see: RADIOLOGICAL TECHNOLOGY

1912 RADIOLOGY UNIT
see: RADIOLOGICAL UNIT

1913 RADIOSCOPY
f radioscopie *f*
e radioscopia *f*
i radioscopia *f*
n radioscopie
d Radioskopie *f*

1914 RADIOSCOPY ROOM
f salle *f* de radioscopie
e sala *f* de radioscopia
i sala *f* di radioscopia
n radioscopieruimte
d Radioskopieraum *m*;
Durchleuchtungsraum *m*

1915 RADIOTHERAP(EUT)IST;
X-RAY THERAP(EUT)IST
f radiothérapeute *m*
e radioterapeuta *m*
i radioterapeuta *m*;
radioterapista *m*
n röntgentherapeut;
radiotherapeut
d Röntgentherapeut *m*

1916 RADIOTHERAPY;
X-RAY THERAPY
f radiothérapie *f*
e radioterapia *f*
i radioterapia *f*
n röntgentherapie;
radiotherapie;
stralentherapie;
bestralingstherapie
d Röntgentherapie *f*;
Strahlentherapie *f*

1917 RADIOTHERAPY CLINIC
f clinique *f* de radiothérapie
e clínica *f* de radioterapia
i clinica *f* di radioterapia
n röntgentherapeutische kliniek;
kliniek voor röntgentherapie
d Klinik *f* für Röntgentherapie;
Klinik *f* für Strahlentherapie

1918 RADIOTHERAPY DEPARTMENT
f service *m* (département *m*) de radiothérapie
e servicio *m* (departamento *m*) de radioterapia
i servizio *m* di radioterapia
n röntgentherapie-afdeling;
radiotherapie-afdeling
d Röntgentherapieabteilung *f*;
Strahlentherapieabteilung *f*

1919 READMISSION
f réadmission *f*
e readmisión *f*
i riaccettazione *f*
n heropneming
d Wiederaufnahme *f*

1920 REANIMATION;
RESUSCITATION
f réanimation *f*
e reanimación *f*;
resucitación *f*
i rianimazione *f*
n reanimatie
d Reanimation *f*

1921 REANIMATION CENTRE (CENTER);
RESUSCITATION CENTRE (CENTER)
f centre *m* de réanimation
e centro *m* de reanimación;
centro *m* de resucitación
i centro *m* di rianimazione
n reanimatiecentrum *n*
d Reanimationszentrum *n*;
Wiederbelebungszentrum *n*

1922 REANIMATION DEPARTMENT;
RESUSCITATION DEPARTMENT
f service *m* (département *m*) de réanimation
e servicio *m* (departamento *m*) de reanimación;
servicio *m* (departamento *m*) de resucitación
i servizio *m* di rianimazione

n reanimatie-afdeling
d Reanimationsabteilung *f*;
Wiederbelebungsabteilung *f*

1923 REANIMATION DOCTOR;
RESUSCITATION DOCTOR
f médecin *m* ressuscitateur
e médico *m* para reanimación;
médico *m* para resucitación
i medico *m* addetto al servizio di rianimazione
n arts voor reanimatie
d Facharzt *m* für Reanimation;
Facharzt *m* für Wiederbelebung

1924 REANIMATION ROOM;
RESUSCITATION ROOM
f salle *f* de réanimation
e sala *f* de reanimación;
sala *f* de resucitación
i sala *f* di rianimazione
n reanimatiekamer
d Reanimationsraum *m*;
Wiederbelebungsraum *m*

1925 REANIMATION UNIT;
RESUSCITATION UNIT
f unité *f* de réanimation
e unidad *f* de reanimación;
unidad *f* de resucitación
i unità *f* di rianimazione
n reanimatie-eenheid
d Reanimationsstation *f*;
Wiederbelebungsstation *f*

1926 RECOVERING PATIENT
see: CONVALESCENT PATIENT

1927 RECOVERY DEPARTMENT
see: POST-ANESTHETIC DEPARTMENT

1928 RECOVERY PATIENT
see: POST-ANESTHETIC PATIENT

1929 RECOVERY ROOM
see: POST-ANESTHETIC ROOM

1930 RECOVERY UNIT
see: POST-ANESTHETIC UNIT

1931 RECTOSCOPY
f rectoscopie *f*
e rectoscopia *f*
i rettoscopia *f*
n rectoscopie
d Rektoskopie *f*

1932 RED CROSS
f Croix *f* Rouge
e Cruz *f* Roja
i Croce *f* Rossa
n Rode Kruis *n*
d Rotes Kreuz *n*

1933 REGIONAL HOSPITAL
f hôpital *m* régional;
hôpital *m* de zone;
centre *m* hospitalier régional
e hospital *m* regional;
hospital *m* comarcal
i ospedale *m* (generale) regionale
n streekziekenhuis *n*
d Regionalkrankenhaus *n*;
Gebietskrankenhaus *n*;
Kreiskrankenhaus *n*;
Bezirkskrankenhaus *n*;
Landesbezirkskrankenhaus *n*

1934 REGIONAL HOSPITAL PLAN
f plan *m* hospitalier régional;
plan *m* régional des hôpitaux
e plan *m* hospitalario regional;
plan *m* regional de hospitales
i piano *m* ospedaliero regionale
n regionaal ziekenhuisplan *n*
d Krankenhausregionalplan *m*

1935 REGISTERED NURSE
see: DIPLOMA NURSE

1936 REGISTRAR
see: CONSULTANT

1937 REHABILITATION
f réadaptation *f*;
révalidation *f*;
réhabilitation *f*;
rééducation *f*
e revalidación *f*;
rehabilitación *f*;
readaptación *f*
i riabilitazione *f*;
rieducazione *f*;
riadattamento *m*;
recupero *m*
n revalidatie;
reactivering
d Rehabilitation *f*

1938 REHABILITATION APPARATUS
f appareils *mpl* de réadaptation
e aparatos *mpl* de revalidación
i apparecchi *mpl* di recupero e rieducazione funzionale
n revalidatie-apparatuur
d Rehabilitationsgeräte *npl*

1939 REHABILITATION BATH
f bain *m* de réadaptation
e baño *m* de revalidación
i bagno *m* per la riabilitazione funzionale
n revalidatiebad *n*
d Rehabilitationsbad *n*

1940 REHABILITATION CENTRE (CENTER)
f centre *m* de réadaptation;
centre *m* de révalidation;
centre *m* de réhabilitation;
centre *m* de rééducation
e centro *m* de revalidación;
centro *m* de rehabilitación;
centro *m* de readaptación
i centro *m* di recupero e di rieducazione funzionale
n revalidatiecentrum *n*
d Rehabilitationszentrum *n*;
Rehabilitierungszentrum *n*

1941 REHABILITATION CLINIC
f clinique *f* de réadaptation;
clinique *f* de révalidation;
clinique *f* de réhabilitation;
clinique *f* de rééducation
e clínica *f* de revalidación;
clínica *f* de rehabilitación;
clínica *f* de readaptación

i clinica *f* di recupero e rieducazione funzionale
n revalidatiekliniek
d Rehabilitationsklinik *f*;
Rehabilitierungsklinik *f*

1942 REHABILITATION DEPARTMENT
f service *m* (département *m*) de réadaptation;
service *m* (département *m*) de révalidation;
service *m* (département *m*) de réhabilitation;
service *m* (département *m*) de rééducation
e servicio *m* (departamento *m*) revalidación
servicio *m* (departamento *m*) de rehabilitación;
servicio *m* (departamento *m*) de readaptación
i servizio *m* di recupero e rieducazione funzionale
n revalidatie-afdeling
d Rehabilitationsabteilung *f*;
Rehabilitierungsabteilung *f*

1943 REHABILITATION HOSPITAL
f hôpital *m* de réadaptation;
hôpital *m* de révalidation;
hôpital *m* de réhabilitation
hôpital *m* de rééducation
e hospital *m* de revalidación;
hospital *m* de rehabilitación;
hospital *m* de readaptación
i ospedale *m* di recupero e rieducazione funzionale
n revalidatieziekenhuis *n*
d Rehabilitationskrankenhaus *n*;
Rehabilitierungskrankenhaus *n*

1944 REHABILITATION INSTITUTION
f établissement *m* de réadaptation;
établissement *m* de révalidation;
établissement *m* de réhabilitation;
établissement *m* de rééducation
e institución *f* de revalidación;
institución *f* de rehabilitación;
institución *f* de readaptación
i stabilimento *m* di recupero e rieducazione funzionale
n revalidatie-inrichting
d Rehabilitationseinrichtung *f*;
Rehabilitierungseinrichtung *f*

1945 REHABILITATION OFFICER;
REHABILITATION SPECIALIST
f médecin *m* de réadaptation;
médecin *m* de révalidation;
médecin *m* de réhabilitation;
médecin *m* de rééducation
e médico *m* rehabilitador;
especialista *m* rehabilitador
i medico *m* della riabilitazione funzionale
n revalidatie-arts
d Rehabilitationsarzt *m*;
Rehabilitierungsarzt *m*

1946 REHABILITATION PROGRAM(ME)
f programme *m* de réadaptation
e plan *m* de revalidación
i programma *m* di recupero e rieducazione funzionale
n revalidatieplan *n*
d Rehabilitationsplan *m*

1947 REHABILITATION SERVICES
f services *mpl* de réadaptation
e servicios *mpl* de revalidación
i servizi *mpl* di recupero e rieducazione funzionale
n revalidatievoorzieningen
d Rehabilitationsdienste *mpl*

1948 REHABILITATION SPECIALIST
see: REHABILITATION OFFICER

1949 REHABILITATION TEAM
f équipe *f* de réadaptation
e equipo *m* de revalidación
i équipe *f* di recupero e rieducazione funzionale
n revalidatieteam *n*
d Rehabilitationsteam *n*

1950 REHABILITATION TREATMENT
f traitement *m* de réadaptation
e tratamiento *m* de revalidación
i trattamento *m* di recupero e rieducazione funzionale
n revalidatiebehandeling
d Rehabilitationsbehandlung *f*

1951 REHABILITATION WORKSHOP
f atelier *m* spécial de réadaptation
e taller *m* de revalidación
i centro *m* speciale di recupero e rieducazione funzionale
n revalidatiewerkplaats
d Rehabilitationswerkstatt *f*;
Rehabilitationswerkstätte *f*

1952 RELIGIOUS HOSPITAL
f hôpital *m* religieux
e hospital *m* religioso
i ospedale *m* religioso
n confessioneel ziekenhuis *n*
d kirchliches Krankenhaus *n*

1953 RELIGIOUS SERVICE
f service *m* des cultes
e servicio *m* religioso
i servizio *m* di assistenza religiosa
n dienst geestelijke verzorging
d Seelsorgedienst *m*

1954 REMEDY
see: DRUG

1955 RENAL DIALYSIS
f dialyse *f* rénale
e diálisis *f* renal
i dialisi *f* renale
n nierdialyse
d Nierendialyse *f*

1956 RENAL DIALYSIS UNIT
f unité *f* de dialyse rénale
e unidad *f* de diálisis renal
i unità *f* di dialisi renale
n nierdialyse-eenheid
d Nierendialysestation *f*

1957 RESEARCH HOSPITAL
f hôpital *m* de recherche
e hospital *m* de investigación
i ospedale *m* di ricerca
n onderzoeksziekenhuis *n*
d Forschungskrankenhaus *n*

1958 RESEARCH LABORATORY
f laboratoire *m* de recherche
e laboratorio *m* de investigación
i laboratorio *m* di ricerca
n onderzoekslaboratorium *n*
d Forschungslaboratorium *n*

1959 RESORT FOR THE AGED
see: GERIATRIC HOME

1960 RESPIRATORY APPARATUS
f appareils *mpl* respiratoires
e aparatos *mpl* respiratorios
i apparecchi *mpl* respiratori
n ademhalingsapparatuur
d Atmungsgeräte *npl*

1961 RESPIRATORY CARE UNIT;
RESPIRATORY UNIT
f unité *f* de soins respiratoires
e unidad *f* de cuidado respiratorio;
unidad *f* de atención respiratoria
i unità *f* di cure respiratorie
n ademhalingsafdeling
d Atmungsabteilung *f*

1962 RESPIRATORY THERAP(EUT)IST
see: INHALATION THERAPEUTIST

1963 RESPIRATORY THERAPY
see: INHALATION THERAPY

1964 RESPIRATORY THERAPY DEPARTMENT
see: INHALATION THERAPY DEPARTMENT

1965 RESPIRATORY UNIT
see: RESPIRATORY CARE UNIT

1966 REST HOME;
RETIREMENT HOME
f maison *f* de retraite;
maison *f* de repos
e casa *f* de reposo
i casa *f* di riposo
n rusthuis *n*
d Erholungsheim *n*

1967 RESUSCITATION
see: REANIMATION

1968 RESUSCITATION CENTRE (CENTER)
see: REANIMATION CENTRE (CENTER)

1969 RESUSCITATION DEPARTMENT
see: REANIMATION DEPARTMENT

1970 RESUSCITATION DOCTOR
see: REANIMATION DOCTOR

1971 RESUSCITATION ROOM
see: REANIMATION ROOM

1972 RESUSCITATION UNIT
see: REANIMATION UNIT

1973 RETIREMENT HOME
see: REST HOME

1974 RHEUMATISM CENTRE (CENTER)
f centre *m* de rhumatologie
e centro *m* de reumatología
i centro *m* di reumatologia
n reumacentrum *n*
d Rheumazentrum *n*

1975 RHEUMATISM CLINIC
f clinique *f* de rhumatologie
e clínica *f* de reumatología
i clinica *f* di reumatologia
n reumakliniek
d Rheumaklinik *f*

1976 RHEUMATISM CONTROL
f lutte *f* contre le rhumatisme
e lucha *f* contra el reumatismo
i lotta *f* contro le malattie reumatiche
n reumabestrijding
d Rheumabekämpfung *f*

1977 RHEUMATISM DEPARTMENT
f service *m* (département *m*) de rhumatologie
e servicio *m* (departamento *m*) de reumatología
i servizio *m* di reumatologia
n reuma-afdeling
d Rheuma-Abteilung *f*

1978 RHEUMATISM UNIT
f unité *f* de rhumatologie
e unidad *f* de reumatología
i unità *f* di reumatologia
n reuma-eenheid
d Rheumastation *f*

1979 RHEUMATOLOGIST
f rhumatologue *m*
e reumatólogo *m*
i reumatologo *m*
n reumatoloog
d Rheumatologe *m*

1980 RHEUMATOLOGY
f rhumatologie *f*
e reumatología *f*
i reumatologia *f*
n reumatologie
d Rheumatologie *f*

1981 ROOM FOR MUD AND WAX BATHS
f salle *f* pour bains de boue et de paraffine
e sala *f* para baños de fango y parafina
i sala *f* per bagni di fango e di paraffina
n ruimte voor modder- en paraffinebaden
d Raum *m* für Schlamm- und Paraffinbäder

1982 ROTATION UNIT
f unité *f* de rotation
e unidad *f* de rotación
i unità *f* di rotazione
n rotatie-eenheid
d Rotationsstation *f*

1983 ROUTINE CARE
f soins *mpl* de routine
e cuidado *m* de rutina;
atención *f* de rutina
i cure *fpl* di routine
n routineverzorging
d Regelversorgung *f*

1984 ROUTINE EXAMINATION
f examen *m* de routine
e examen *m* de rutina
i esame *m* di routine
n routine-onderzoek *n*
d Routineuntersuchung *f*

1985 ROUTINE LABORATORY
f laboratoire *m* de routine
e laboratorio *m* de rutina
i laboratorio *m* per analisi di routine
n routinelaboratorium *n*
d Routinelaboratorium *n*

1986 RURAL HEALTH CARE FACILITIES;
RURAL HEALTH CARE SERVICES;
RURAL HEALTH FACILITIES;
RURAL HEALTH SERVICES

f services *mpl* sanitaires ruraux;
services *mpl* de santé ruraux

e servicios *mpl* sanitarios rurales;
servicios *mpl* de salud rurales;
servicios *mpl* de sanidad rurales

i servizi *mpl* sanitari rurali

n gezondheidsvoorzieningen op het platteland;
gezondheidsdiensten op het platteland

d Gesundheitsfürsorgedienste *mpl* in ländlichen Gebieten;
Gesundheitswesen *n* in ländlichen Gebieten

1987 RURAL HEALTH CARE SERVICES
see: RURAL HEALTH CARE FACILITIES

1988 RURAL HEALTH FACILITIES
see: RURAL HEALTH CARE FACILITIES

1989 RURAL HEALTH SERVICES
see: RURAL HEALTH CARE FACILITIES

1990 RURAL HOSPITAL
see: COTTAGE HOSPITAL

S

1991 SANATORIUM
f sanatorium *m*;
maison *f* de cure
e sanatorio *m*;
casa *f* de salud
i sanatorio *m*;
casa *f* di cura
n sanatorium *n*
d Sanatorium *n*;
Heilstätte *f*;
Heilanstalt *f*;
Kuranstalt *f*;
Kureinrichtung *f*

1992 SANITARY APPARATUS
f appareils *mpl* sanitaires
e aparatos *mpl* sanitarios
i apparecchi *mpl* sanitari
n sanitaire apparatuur
d Sanitärgeräte *npl*

1993 SANITARY ECONOMICS
see: HEALTH ECONOMICS

1994 SANITARY ECONOMIST
see: HEALTH ECONOMIST

1995 SANITARY EDUCATION
see: HEALTH EDUCATION

1996 SANITARY EQUIPMENT
f installations *fpl* sanitaires
e instalaciones *fpl* sanitarias
i installazioni *fpl* sanitarie
n sanitair *n*
d sanitäre Anlagen *fpl*;
sanitäre Einrichtungen *fpl*

1997 SANITARY INSTITUTION
see: HEALTH CARE INSTITUTION

1998 SANITARY ORGANIZATION
see: HEALTH CARE ORGANIZATION

1999 SANITARY PLANNING
see: HEALTH CARE PLANNING

2000 SANITARY PROTECTION
see: HEALTH PROTECTION

2001 SANITARY REFORM
see: HEALTH REFORM

2002 SANITARY REGULATION
f règlement *m* sanitaire
e prescripción *f* sanitaria
i regolamento *m* sanitario
n gezondheidsvoorschrift *n*
d Gesundheitsvorschrift *f*

2003 SCHOOL DENTAL CARE;
SCHOOL DENTAL HEALTH CARE
f soins *mpl* dentaires dans les écoles
e asistencia *f* dental escolar
i cure *fpl* dentarie nelle scuole
n schooltandverzorging
d Schulzahnpflege *f*

2004 SCHOOL DENTAL HEALTH CARE
see: SCHOOL DENTAL CARE

2005 SCHOOL DOCTOR;
SCHOOL MEDICAL OFFICER;
SCHOOL PHYSICIAN
f médecin *m* scolaire;
médecin *m* des écoles
e médico *m* escolar
i medico *m* scolare
n schoolarts
d Schularzt *m*

2006 SCHOOL FOR NURSES
see: NURSES' SCHOOL

2007 SCHOOL FOR NURSING
see: NURSES' SCHOOL

2008 SCHOOL HEALTH CARE
f soins *mpl* sanitaires dans les écoles
e cuidado *m* sanitario escolar
i assistenza *f* sanitaria nelle scuole
n schoolgezondheidszorg
d Schulgesundheitspflege *f*

2009 SCHOOL HEALTH NURSE;
SCHOOL NURSE
f infirmière *f* scolaire
e enfermera *f* escolar
i infermiera *f* scolare
n schoolverpleegster
d Schulpflegerin *f*

2010 SCHOOL HEALTH SERVICE
f service *m* sanitaire scolaire
e servicio *m* sanitario escolar
i servizio *m* sanitario scolastico
n schoolartsendienst;
geneeskundig schooltoezicht *n*
d Schulgesundheitsdienst *m*

2011 SCHOOL HYGIENE
f hygiène *f* scolaire
e higiene *f* escolar
i igiene *f* scolare
n schoolhygiëne
d Schulhygiene *f*

2012 SCHOOL MEDICAL OFFICER
see: SCHOOL DOCTOR

2013 SCHOOL MEDICINE
f médecine *f* scolaire
e medicina *f* escolar
i medicina *f* scolare
n schoolgeneeskunde
d Schulmedizin *f*

2014 SCHOOL NURSE
see: SCHOOL HEALTH NURSE

2015 SCHOOL OF NURSING
see: NURSES' SCHOOL

2016 SCHOOL PHYSICIAN
see: SCHOOL DOCTOR

2017 SCIENCE OF NURSING
see: NURSING SCIENCE

2018 SCIENTIFIC MEDICINE
f médecine *f* scientifique
e medicina *f* científica
i medicina *f* scientifica
n wetenschappelijke geneeskunde
d wissenschaftliche Medizin *f*

2019 SCOTCH SHOWER
f douche *f* écossaise
e ducha *f* escocesa
i doccia *f* scozzese
n Schotse douche
d schottische Dusche *f*

2020 SELF CARE
f autosoins *mpl*
e auto-cuidado *m*
i autocure *fpl*
n zelfverzorging
d Selbstpflege *f*

2021 SELF CARE UNIT
f unité *f* d'autosoins
e unidad *f* de auto-cuidado
i unità *f* d'autocure
n zelfverzorgingseenheid
d Selbstpflegestation *f*

2022 SEMI-PUBLIC HOSPITAL
f hôpital *m* semi-public
e hospital *m* semi-público
i ospedale *m* semi-pubblico
n semi-openbaar ziekenhuis *n*;
semi-overheidsziekenhuis *n*
d halb-öffentliches Krankenhaus *n*

2023 SENSORIAL HANDICAP
f déficience *f* sensorielle
e impedimento *m* sensorial
i deficienza *f* sensoriale
n zintuiglijke handicap
d sinnliche Behinderung *f*

2024 SEPTIC PATIENT
f malade *m* (patient *m*) septique
e paciente *m* (enfermo *m*) séptico
i malato *m* settico
n septische patiënt
d septischer Patient *m* (Kranker *m*)

2025 SEQUENCE OF CARE
f succession *f* des soins
e orden *m/f* de cuidado (atención)
i successione *f* delle cure
n volgorde van verzorging
d Pflegefolge *f*

2026 SERIOUSLY HANDICAPPED;
SEVERELY HANDICAPPED
f grand infirme *m*;
grand mutilé *m*
e gran mutilado *m*;
grave mutilado *m*
i grande invalido *m*;
grande mutilato *m*
n zwaar gehandicapte;
ernstig gehandicapte
d Schwerbehinderter *m*;
Schwerbeschädigter *m*

2027 SEVERELY HANDICAPPED
see: SERIOUSLY HANDICAPPED

2028 SEVERELY ILL PATIENT
f grand malade *m*
e grave enfermo *m*
i malato *m* grave
n ernstig zieke patiënt
d schwerer Kranker *m*

2029 SEVERE MENTAL DEFICIENCY;
SEVERE MENTAL RETARDATION
f faiblesse *f* mentale profonde;
déficience *f* mentale profonde;
débilité *f* mentale profonde
e deficiencia *f* mental grave;
debilidad *f* mental grave;
disminución *f* mental grave;
minusvalía *f* mental grave
i debolezza *f* mentale profonda;
deficienza *f* mentale profonda
n diepe zwakzinnigheid
d tiefe Geistesschwäche *f*;
tiefer Schwachsinn *m*;
tiefe geistige Behinderung *f*

2030 SEVERE MENTAL RETARDATION
see: SEVERE MENTAL DEFICIENCY

2031 SHELTERED EMPLOYMENT
see: PROTECTED EMPLOYMENT

2032 SHELTERED WORK
see: PROTECTED EMPLOYMENT

2033 SHELTERED WORKSHOP
see: PROTECTED WORKSHOP

2034 SHIP'S DOCTOR;
SHIP'S SURGEON
f médecin *m* de bord
e médico *m* de a bordo;
médico *m* del barco
i medico *m* di bordo
n scheepsdokter;
scheepsarts
d Schiffsarzt *m*

2035 SHIP'S SURGEON
see: SHIP'S DOCTOR

2036 SHORTAGE OF NURSES
see: NURSING SHORTAGE

2037 SHORT STAY CARE;
SHORT STAY PATIENT CARE;
SHORT TERM CARE;
SHORT TERM PATIENT CARE
f soins *mpl* de courte durée
e cuidado *m* (atención *f*) a corto plazo
i cure *fpl* di breve durata
n zorg voor kortstondig zieken
d Kurzzeitpflege *f*;
kurzfristige Pflege *f*

2038 SHORT STAY HOSPITAL;
SHORT TERM HOSPITAL
f hôpital *m* de court séjour;
hôpital *m* à court terme
e hospital *m* de corto plazo
i ospedale *m* generale
n algemeen ziekenhuis *n*
d Akutkrankenhaus *n*;
Kurzaufenthaltskrankenhaus *n*

2039 SHORT STAY HOSPITAL CARE;
SHORT TERM HOSPITAL CARE
f soins *mpl* hospitaliers de courte durée
e cuidado *m* hospitalario a corto plazo;
atención *f* hospitalaria a corto plazo
i cure *fpl* ospedaliere di breve durata
n kortstondige ziekenhuisverpleging
d kurzfristige Krankenhauspflege *f*

2040 SHORT STAY PATIENT CARE
see: SHORT STAY CARE

2041 SHORT TERM CARE
see: SHORT STAY CARE

2042 SHORT TERM HOSPITAL
see: SHORT STAY HOSPITAL

2043 SHORT TERM HOSPITAL CARE
see: SHORT STAY HOSPITAL CARE

2044 SHORT TERM PATIENT CARE
see: SHORT STAY CARE

2045 SHORT TERM THERAPY
f thérapie *f* de courte durée
e terapia *f* a corto plazo
i terapia *f* di breve durata
n kortdurende therapie
d kurzfristige Therapie *f*

2046 SICK ABSENTEEISM
see: ABSENCE DUE TO SICKNESS

2047 SICK-BAY;
SICK-BERTH
f poste *m* des malades
e camarote *m* para enfermos
i posto *m* dei malati
n ziekenboeg
d Krankenverschlag *m*;
Krankenkoje *f*;
Krankenkajüte *f*

2048 SICK-BED
f lit *m* de malade
e cama *f* de enfermo;
lecho *m* de enfermo
i letto *m* d'ammalato
n ziekbed *n*
d Krankenbett *n*

2049 SICK BENEFIT;
SICK PAY
f indemnité *f* de maladie
e subsidio *m* de enfermedad;
pago *m* del seguro de enfermedad
i indennità *f* di malattia
n ziekengeld *n*
d Krankengeld *n*

2050 SICK-BERTH
see: SICK-BAY

2051 SICK-FUND
see: HEALTH INSURANCE FUND

2052 SICK-FUND MEMBER;
SOCIAL INSURANCE PATIENT
f malade *m* (patient *m*) assuré social
e paciente *m* (enfermo *m*) de la caja de enfermedad
i malato *m* avente un'assicurazione sociale
n (zieken)fondsverzekerde;
(zieken)fondspatiënt
d Kassenpatient *m*;
Krankenkassenpatient *m*

2053 SICK-LEAVE
f congé *m* de maladie;
congé *m* de convalescence;
congé *m* pour raisons de santé
e licencia *f* de convalecencia
i congedo *m* di convalescenza
n ziekteverlof *n*
d Krankheitsurlaub *m*;
Krankenurlaub *m*

2054 SICKNESS
see: DISEASE

2055 SICKNESS ABSENCE
see: ABSENCE DUE TO SICKNESS

2056 SICKNESS ABSENTEEISM
see: ABSENCE DUE TO SICKNESS

2057 SICKNESS COSTS INSURANCE
see: HEALTH CARE INSURANCE

2058 SICKNESS INSURANCE
see: HEALTH CARE INSURANCE

2059 SICK PAY
see: SICK BENEFIT

2060 SICK-RATE
see: MORBIDITY

2061 SICK ROOM
see: PATIENT ROOM

2062 SICK WARD
see: HOSPITAL WARD

2063 SISTER
see: CHIEF NURSE

2064 SKIN BANK
f banque *f* de peau
e banco *m* de piel
i banca *f* della pelle
n huidbank
d Hautbank *f*

2065 SKIN DISEASES CLINIC
see: DERMATOLOGY CLINIC

2066 SKIN DISEASES DEPARTMENT
see: DERMATOLOGY DEPARTMENT

2067 SKIN DISEASES HOSPITAL
see: DERMATOLOGY HOSPITAL

2068 SKIN DISEASES UNIT
see: DERMATOLOGY UNIT

2069 SKIN SPECIALIST
see: DERMATOLOGIST

2070 SLEEP TREATMENT
f cure *f* de sommeil
e cura *f* de sueño
i cura *f* del sonno
n slaapkuur
d Schlafkur *f*

2071 SLEEP TREATMENT ROOM
f chambre *f* pour cure de sommeil
e sala *f* de cura de sueño
i camera *f* per la cura del sonno
n slaapkuurkamer
d Raum *m* für Schlafkuren

2072 SMALL HOSPITAL
f petit hôpital *m*
e hospital *m* menor
i ospedale *m* piccolo
n klein ziekenhuis *n*
d Kleinkrankenhaus *n*

2073 SMALLPOX DEPARTMENT
f service *m* (département *m*) pour varioleux
e servicio *m* (departamento *m*) de viruela
i servizio *m* antivaioloso
n pokkenafdeling
d Pockenabteilung *f*

2074 SOCIAL AID;
SOCIAL ASSISTANCE;
SOCIAL WORK
f assistance *f* sociale;
aide *f* sociale;
travail *m* social
e asistencia *f* social;
ayuda *f* social;
trabajo *m* social
i assistenza *f* sociale;
lavoro *m* sociale
n maatschappelijk werk *n*
d soziale Fürsorge *f*;
Sozialhilfe *f*;
soziale Hilfe *f*;
Sozialarbeit *f*;
Sozialbetreuung *f*

2075 SOCIAL ASSISTANCE
see: SOCIAL AID

2076 SOCIAL GERONTOLOGIST
f gérontologiste *m* social;
gérontologue *m* social
e gerontólogo *m* social
i gerontologo *m* sociale
n sociaal gerontoloog
d Sozialgerontologe *m*

2077 SOCIAL GERONTOLOGY
f gérontologie *f* sociale
e gerontología *f* social
i gerontologia *f* sociale
n sociale gerontologie
d Sozialgerontologie *f*

2078 SOCIAL HEALTH CARE INSURANCE;
SOCIAL HEALTH (COSTS) INSURANCE;
SOCIAL SICKNESS (COSTS) INSURANCE
f assurance-maladie *f* sociale;
assurance *f* sociale contre la maladie
e seguro *m* de enfermedad social;
seguro *m* de salud social
i assicurazione *f* sociale contro le malattie
n sociale verzekering tegen ziektekosten
d soziale Krankenversicherung *f*

2079 SOCIAL HEALTH COSTS INSURANCE
see: SOCIAL HEALTH CARE INSURANCE

2080 SOCIAL HEALTH INSURANCE
see: SOCIAL HEALTH CARE INSURANCE

2081 SOCIAL INSURANCE
f assurance *f* sociale
e seguro *m* social
i assicurazione *f* sociale
n sociale verzekering
d Sozialversicherung *f*

2082 SOCIAL INSURANCE INSTITUTION
f institution *f* d'assurance sociale
e institución *f* de seguro social;
organismo *m* de seguro social
i istituto *m* d'assicurazione sociale
n uitvoeringsorgaan *n* van de sociale verzekering
d Sozialversicherungsträger *m*

2083 SOCIAL INSURANCE MEDICINE
f médecine *f* d'assurance sociale
e medicina *f* de seguro social
i medicina *f* d'assicurazione sociale
n sociale verzekeringsgeneeskunde
d Sozialversicherungsmedizin *f*

2084 SOCIAL INSURANCE PATIENT
see: SICK-FUND MEMBER

2085 SOCIAL MEDICINE
f médecine *f* sociale
e medicina *f* social
i medicina *f* sociale
n sociale geneeskunde
d Sozialmedizin *f*;
soziale Medizin *f*

2086 SOCIAL MEDICINE DEPARTMENT
f service *m* (département *m*) de médecine sociale
e servicio *m* (departamento *m*) de medicina social
i servizio *m* di medicina sociale
n sociaal-geneeskundige afdeling
d sozialmedizinische Abteilung *f*

2087 SOCIAL MEDICINE HOSPITAL
f hôpital *m* de médecine sociale
e hospital *m* de medicina social
i ospedale *m* per le malattie sociali
n ziekenhuis *n* voor sociale geneeskunde
d Krankenhaus *n* für Sozialmedizin

2088 SOCIAL MEDICINE UNIT
f unité *f* de médecine sociale
e unidad *f* de medicina social
i unità *f* di medicina sociale
n sociaal-geneeskundige eenheid
d sozialmedizinische Station *f*

2089 SOCIAL PSYCHIATRY
f psychiatrie *f* sociale
e psiquiatría *f* social
i psichiatria *f* sociale
n sociale psychiatrie
d Sozialpsychiatrie *f*;
soziale Psychiatrie *f*

2090 SOCIAL SECURITY
f sécurité *f* sociale
e seguridad *f* social
i sicurezza *f* sociale
n sociale zekerheid
d soziale Sicherheit *f*

2091 SOCIAL SICKNESS COSTS INSURANCE
see: SOCIAL HEALTH CARE INSURANCE

2092 SOCIAL SICKNESS INSURANCE
see: SOCIAL HEALTH CARE INSURANCE

2093 SOCIAL THERAPY;
SOCIOTHERAPY
f thérapie *f* sociale;
sociothérapie *f*
e terapia *f* social;
socioterapia *f*
i terapia *f* sociale;
socioterapia *f*
n sociale therapie;
sociotherapie
d Sozialtherapie *f*;
soziale Therapie *f*

2094 SOCIAL THERAPY CENTRE (CENTER);
SOCIOTHERAPY CENTRE (CENTER)
f centre *m* sociothérapeutique;
centre *m* de sociothérapie
e centro *m* socioterapéutico;
centro *m* de socioterapia
i centro *m* socioterapico;
centro *m* di socioterapia
n sociotherapeutisch centrum *n*
d sozialtherapeutisches Zentrum *n*

2095 SOCIAL WORK
see: SOCIAL AID

2096 SOCIAL WORKER
f assistant *m* social;
travailleur *m* social
e asistente *m* social;
trabajador *m* social
i assistente *m* sociale;
operatore *m* sociale
n maatschappelijk werker;
sociaal werker
d Sozialfürsorger *m*;
Sozialarbeiter *m*

2097 SOCIO-PSYCHIATRIC CARE
f soins *mpl* socio-psychiatriques
e cuidado *m* social psiquiátrico
i cure *fpl* di psichiatria sociale
n sociaal-psychiatrische zorg
d sozialpsychiatrische Versorgung *f*

2098 SOCIO-PSYCHIATRIC SERVICE
f service *m* socio-psychiatrique
e servicio *m* social psiquiátrico
i servizio *m* di psichiatria sociale
n sociaal-psychiatrische dienst;
S.P.D.
d sozialpsychiatrischer Dienst *m*

2099 SOCIOTHERAPY
see: SOCIAL THERAPY

2100 SOCIOTHERAPY CENTRE (CENTER)
see: SOCIAL THERAPY CENTRE (CENTER)

2101 SOMATIC DISEASE
see: PHYSICAL DISEASE

2102 SOMATIC HEALTH CARE
see: PHYSICAL HEALTH CARE

2103 SOMATIC HOSPITAL
f hôpital *m* pour malades somatiques
e hospital *m* para enfermedades somáticas
i ospedale *m* per le malattie somatiche
n ziekenhuis *n* voor somatische patiënten
d Krankenhaus *n* für somatische Patienten

2104 SOMATIC ILLNESS
see: PHYSICAL DISEASE

2105 SOMATIC PATIENT
see: PHYSICAL PATIENT

2106 SPECIAL CARE;
SPECIALIZED CARE
f soins *mpl* spéciaux;
soins *mpl* spécialisés
e cuidado *m* especialista;
atención *f* (asistencia *f*) especialista
i cure *fpl* specialistiche
n specialistische hulp
d Fachpflege *f*;
Sonderpflege *f*;
Spezialpflege *f*

2107 SPECIAL DEPARTMENT;
SPECIALIZED DEPARTMENT
f service *m* (département *m*) spécialisé
e servicio *m* (departamento *m*) especializado
i servizio *m* specialistico
n specialistische afdeling
d Fachabteilung *f*;
Sonderabteilung *f*;
Spezialabteilung *f*

2108 SPECIAL DUTY NURSE
f infirmière *f* spécialisée
e enfermera *f* especialista
i infermiera *f* specializzata
n gespecialiseerde verpleegkundige
d Sonderkrankenpflegerin *f*

2109 SPECIAL HOSPITAL;
SPECIALIZED HOSPITAL
f hôpital *m* spécialisé;
établissement *m* hospitalier spécialisé
e hospital *m* especializado
i ospedale *m* specializzato
n categoraal ziekenhuis *n*;
speciaal ziekenhuis *n*
d Fachkrankenhaus *n*;
Sonderkrankenhaus *n*;
Spezialkrankenhaus *n*

2110 SPECIAL HOSPITAL BED;
SPECIALIZED HOSPITAL BED
f lit *m* hospitalier spécial;
lit *m* hospitalier spécialisé
e cama *f* hospitalaria especializada
i letto *m* d'ospedale specializzato
n specialistisch ziekenhuisbed *n*
d spezialisiertes Krankenhausbett *n*

2111 SPECIALIST
see: CONSULTANT

2112 SPECIALIZED CARE
see: SPECIAL CARE

2113 SPECIALIZED DEPARTMENT
see: SPECIAL DEPARTMENT

2114 SPECIALIZED HOSPITAL
see: SPECIAL HOSPITAL

2115 SPECIALIZED HOSPITAL BED
see: SPECIAL HOSPITAL BED

2116 SPECIALIZED SERVICES;
SPECIAL SERVICES
f services *mpl* spéciaux;
services *mpl* spécialisés
e servicios *mpl* especialistas;
servicios *mpl* especializados
i servizi *mpl* specialistici
n specialistische diensten
d fachärztliche Dienste *mpl*

2117 SPECIALIZED UNIT;
SPECIAL UNIT
f unité *f* spécialisée
e unidad *f* especializada
i unità *f* specialistica
n specialistische eenheid
d Fachstation *f*;
Sonderstation *f*;
Spezialstation *f*

2118 SPECIAL NURSING;
SPECIAL NURSING CARE
f soins *mpl* infirmiers spéciaux;
soins *mpl* infirmiers spécialisés
e enfermería *f* especialista;
cuidado *m* enfermero especialista;
atención *f* (asistencia *f*) enfermera especialista
i cure *fpl* infermieristiche specialistiche
n specialistische verpleging
d Sonderkrankenpflege *f*

2119 SPECIAL NURSING CARE
see: SPECIAL NURSING

2120 SPECIAL NURSING DEPARTMENT
f service *m* (département *m*) de soins infirmiers spéciaux
e servicio *m* (departamento *m*) de enfermería especialista
i divisione *f* di cure infermieristiche specialistiche
n gespecialiseerde verpleegafdeling
d Sonderpflegeabteilung *f*

2121 SPECIAL NURSING UNIT
f unité *f* de soins infirmiers spéciaux
e unidad *f* de enfermería especialista
i unità *f* di cure infermieristiche specialistiche
n gespecialiseerde verpleegeenheid
d Sonderpflegestation *f*

2122 SPECIAL SCHOOL FOR THE HANDICAPPED
f école *f* spécialisée pour handicapés
e escuela *f* especializada para impedidos
i scuola *f* specializzata per handicappati
n mytylschool
d Sonderschule *f* für Behinderte

2123 SPECIAL SERVICES
see: SPECIALIZED SERVICES

2124 SPECIAL SURGEON
f chirurgien *m* spécialisé
e cirujano *m* especialista
i chirurgo *m* specializzato
n gespecialiseerd chirurg
d Fachchirurg *m*

2125 SPECIAL SURGERY
f chirurgie *f* spécialisée
e cirugía *f* especialista
i chirurgia *f* specializzata
n specialistische chirurgie
d Fachchirurgie *f*

2126 SPECIAL SURGERY DEPARTMENT
f service *m* (département *m*) de chirurgie spécialisée
e servicio *m* (departamento *m*) de cirugía especialista
i servizio *m* di chirurgia specializzata
n specialistische chirurgische afdeling
d chirurgische Fachabteilung *f*

2127 SPECIAL THERAPY
f thérapie *f* spéciale
e terapia *f* especial
i terapia *f* speciale
n speciale therapie
d Sondertherapie *f*

2128 SPECIAL UNIT
see: SPECIALIZED UNIT

2129 SPECIMEN COLLECTING ROOM;
SPECIMEN TAKING ROOM
f salle *f* de prélèvement
e sala *f* para hacer especímenes
i sala *f* per prelievi
n prikkamer
d Raum *m* für Entnahme von Untersuchungsgut

2130 SPECIMEN TAKING ROOM
see: SPECIMEN COLLECTING ROOM

2131 SPEECH THERAPY
see: LOGOPEDICS

2132 SPEECH THERAPY DEPARTMENT
see: LOGOPEDICS DEPARTMENT

2133 SPERM BANK
f banque *f* de sperme
e banco *m* de esperma
i banca *f* dello sperma
n spermabank
d Spermabank *f*

2134 SPORTS MEDICINE
f médecine *f* sportive
e medicina *f* de deporte
i medicina *f* sportiva
n sportgeneeskunde
d Sportmedizin *f*

2135 SPORTS MEDICINE DOCTOR
f médecin *m* de sport
e médico *m* de deporte
i medico *m* sportivo
n sportarts
d Sportarzt *m*

2136 STAFF HEALTH CARE
see: PERSONNEL HEALTH CARE

2137 STAFF HEALTH SERVICE
see: PERSONNEL HEALTH SERVICE

2138 STAFF/PATIENT RATE
see: PERSONNEL/PATIENT RATE

2139 STAFF/PATIENT RATIO
see: PERSONNEL/PATIENT RATE

2140 STAY LENGTH
see: DURATION OF HOSPITALIZATION

2141 STEREOTAXIS ROOM
f salle *f* de stéréotaxie
e sala *f* de estereotaxia
i sala *f* di stereotassia
n stereotaxiekamer
d Stereotaxieraum *m*

2142 STERILE CLOTHING ROOM
f dépôt *m* de vêtements stériles
e almacén *m* de vestidos estériles
i deposito *m* dei vestiti sterilizzati
n berging voor steriele kleding
d Lager *n* für sterile Kleidung

2143 STERILE DRESSING DISTRIBUTION
f distribution *f* de pansements stériles
e distribución *f* de venda estéril
i distribuzione *f* di bende sterili
n uitgifte van steriel verband
d Ausgabe *f* von sterilem Verbandsmaterial

2144 STERILE FLUIDS DEPARTMENT
f service *m* (département *m*) des liquides stériles
e servicio *m* (departamento *m*) de líquidos estériles
i servizio *m* dei liquidi sterili
n steriele vloeistoffen afdeling
d sterile Flüssigkeiten Abteilung *f*

2145 STERILE INSTRUMENTS STORE
f dépôt *m* d'instruments stériles
e almacén *m* de instrumentos estériles
i deposito *m* dei strumenti sterilizzati
n berging voor steriele instrumenten
d Lager *n* für sterile Instrumente

2146 STERILE LINEN
f linge *m* stérile
e ropa *f* estéril
i biancheria *f* sterile
n steriele was
d sterile Wäsche *f*

2147 STERILE STORE
f dépôt *m* de matériel stérile;
dépôt *m* stérile
e almacén *m* de material estéril
i deposito *m* del materiale sterilizzato
n berging voor steriel materiaal;
steriele berging
d Lager *n* für steriles Material

2148 STERILIZABLE BLANKET
f couverture *f* stérilisable
e cobertura *f* esterilizable
i coperta *f* sterilizzabile
n steriliseerbare deken
d sterilisierbare Decke *f*

2149 STERILIZATION APPARATUS;
STERILIZING APPARATUS
f appareils *mpl* de stérilisation
e aparatos *mpl* esterilizadores
i apparecchi *mpl* di sterilizzazione
n sterilisatie-apparatuur
d Sterilisiergeräte *npl*

2150 STERILIZATION DEPARTMENT;
STERILIZING DEPARTMENT
f service *m* (département *m*) de stérilisation
e servicio *m* (departamento *m*) de esterilización
i servizio *m* di sterilizzazione
n sterilisatie-afdeling
d Sterilisationsabteilung *f*

2151 STERILIZATION ROOM;
STERILIZING ROOM
f salle *f* de stérilisation
e sala *f* de esterilización
i sala *f* di sterilizzazione
n sterilisatiekamer
d Sterilisationsraum *m*

2152 STERILIZER
f étuve *f* à stériliser
e esterilizador *m*
i stufa *f* di sterilizzazione
n sterilisator
d Sterilisationsgerät *n*

2153 STERILIZING APPARATUS
see: STERILIZATION APPARATUS

2154 STERILIZING DEPARTMENT
see: STERILIZATION DEPARTMENT

2155 STERILIZING ROOM
see: STERILIZATION ROOM

2156 STOMATOLOGY
f stomatologie *f*
e estomatología *f*
i stomatologia *f*
n stomatologie;
mondheelkunde
d Stomatologie *f*;
Mundheilkunde *f*

2157 STOMATOLOGY DEPARTMENT
f service *m* (département *m*) stomatologique;
service *m* (département *m*) de stomatologie
e servicio *m* (departamento *m*) estomatológico;
servicio *m* (departamento *m*) de estomatología
i divisione *f* di stomatologia
n stomatologische afdeling
d Mundheilkundige Abteilung *f*

2158 STOMATOLOGY HOSPITAL
f hôpital *m* stomatologique;
hôpital *m* de stomatologie
e hospital *m* estomatológico;
hospital *m* de estomatología
i ospedale *m* stomatologico
n ziekenhuis *n* voor stomatologie
d Krankenhaus *n* für Mundheilkunde

2159 STOMATOLOGY UNIT
f unité *f* stomatologique;
unité *f* de stomatologie
e unidad *f* estomatológica;
unidad *f* de estomatología
i unità *f* di stomatologia
n stomatologische eenheid
d Mundheilkundige Station *f*

2160 STRETCHER
f brancard *m*;
civière *f*
e camilla *f*;
angarillas *fpl*;
parihuelas *fpl*
i barella *f*
n brancard
d Tragbahre *f*;
Krankenbahre *f*;
Krankentrage *f*

2161 STRETCHER ROOM
f emplacement *m* pour brancards
e depósito *m* para camillas
i deposito *m* per barelle
n brancardberging
d Abstellraum *m* für Tragbahren

2162 STUDENT DOCTOR
see: MEDICAL STUDENT

2163 STUDENT HEALTH CARE SERVICE;
STUDENT HEALTH SERVICE
f service *m* sanitaire pour étudiants
e servicio *m* sanitario para estudiantes
i servizio *m* di medicina scolare
n gezondheidsdienst voor studenten
d Gesundheitsfürsorgedienst *m* für Studenten

2164 STUDENT HEALTH SERVICE
see: STUDENT HEALTH CARE SERVICE

2165 STUDENT NURSE
see: NURSING STUDENT

2166 SUB-INTENSIVE CARE
f soins *mpl* sous-intensifs
e cuidado *m* subintensivo;
atención *f* subintensiva
i cure *fpl* meno intensive
n subintensieve zorg
d Subintensivpflege *f*

2167 SUPER-SPECIALITY
f super-spécialité *f*
e superespecialidad *f*
i super-specialità *f*
n superspecialisme *n*
d Superspezialität *f*

2168 SUPER-SPECIALIZATION
f super-spécialisation *f*
e superespecialización *f*
i super-specializzazione *f*
n superspecialisatie
d Superspezialisierung *f*

2169 SURGEON
f chirurgien *m*
e cirujano *m*
i chirurgo *m*
n chirurg
d Chirurg *m*

2170 SURGEON DENTIST
see: DENTAL SURGEON

2171 SURGERY
f chirurgie *f*
e cirugía *f*
i chirurgia *f*
n chirurgie
d Chirurgie *f*

2172 SURGERY BLOCK
see: OPERATING BLOCK

2173 SURGERY CENTRE (CENTER);
SURGICAL CENTRE (CENTER)
f centre *m* chirurgical;
centre *m* de chirurgie
e centro *m* quirúrgico;
centro *m* de cirugía
i centro *m* chirurgico;
centro *m* di chirurgia
n chirurgisch centrum *n*
d chirurgisches Zentrum *n*

2174 SURGERY CLINIC;
SURGICAL CLINIC
f clinique *f* chirurgicale;
clinique *f* de chirurgie
e clínica *f* quirúrgica;
clínica *f* de cirugía
i clinica *f* chirurgica
n chirurgische kliniek
d chirurgische Klinik *f*

2175 SURGERY DEPARTMENT
see: OPERATING BLOCK

2176 SURGERY HOSPITAL;
SURGICAL HOSPITAL
f hôpital *m* chirurgical;
hôpital *m* de chirurgie
e hospital *m* quirúrgico;
hospital *m* de cirugía
i ospedale *m* chirurgico
n chirurgisch ziekenhuis *n*
d chirurgisches Krankenhaus *n*

2177 SURGERY SUITE
see: OPERATING BLOCK

2178 SURGERY UNIT;
SURGICAL UNIT
f unité *f* chirurgicale;
unité *f* de chirurgie
e unidad *f* quirúrgica;
unidad *f* de cirugía
i unità *f* chirurgica;
unità *f* di chirurgia
n chirurgische eenheid
d chirurgische Station *f*

2179 SURGICAL ADMISSION
f admission *f* chirurgicale
e admisión *f* quirúrgica
i ammissione *f* chirurgica
n chirurgische opname
d chirurgische Aufnahme *f*

2180 SURGICAL APPARATUS
f appareils *mpl* chirurgicaux

e aparatos *mpl* quirúrgicos
i apparecchi *mpl* chirurgici
n chirurgische apparatuur
d chirurgische Geräte *npl*

2181 SURGICAL BED
f lit *m* chirurgical;
lit *m* de chirurgie
e cama *f* quirúrgica;
cama *f* de cirugía
i letto *m* chirurgico;
letto *m* di chirurgia
n chirurgisch bed *n*
d chirurgisches Bett *n*

2182 SURGICAL BLOCK
see: OPERATING BLOCK

2183 SURGICAL CENTRE (CENTER)
see: SURGERY CENTRE (CENTER)

2184 SURGICAL CLINIC
see: SURGERY CLINIC

2185 SURGICAL CLOTHING
see: OPERATING ROOM CLOTHING

2186 SURGICAL DEPARTMENT
see: OPERATING BLOCK

2187 SURGICAL EXAMINATION
f examen *m* chirurgical
e examen *m* quirúrgico
i esame *m* chirurgico
n chirurgisch onderzoek *n*
d chirurgische Untersuchung *f*

2188 SURGICAL HOSPITAL
see: SURGERY HOSPITAL

2189 SURGICAL INSTRUMENTS
f instruments *mpl* chirurgicaux
e instrumentos *mpl* quirúrgicos
i strumenti *mpl* chirurgici
n chirurgische instrumenten
d chirurgische Instrumente *npl*

2190 SURGICAL INTENSIVE CARE
f soins *mpl* intensifs chirurgicaux
e cuidado *m* intensivo quirúrgico
i cure *fpl* intensive chirurgiche
n chirurgische intensieve zorg
d chirurgische Intensivpflege *f*

2191 SURGICAL LINEN
see: OPERATING ROOM LINEN

2192 SURGICAL NURSING
f soins *mpl* infirmiers chirurgicaux
e enfermería *f* quirúrgica
i cure *fpl* infermieristiche chirurgiche
n chirurgische verpleging
d chirurgische Krankenpflege *f*

2193 SURGICAL OPERATION
see: OPERATION

2194 SURGICAL OUTPATIENT DEPARTMENT
f service *m* (département *m*) de consultations externes de chirurgie
e servicio *m* (departamento *m*) de consultas externas de cirugía
i consultorio *m* di chirurgia
n chirurgische polikliniek
d chirurgisches Ambulatorium *n*

2195 SURGICAL PATIENT
f malade *m* (patient *m*) chirurgical;
malade *m* (patient *m*) de chirurgie
e paciente *m* (enfermo *m*) quirúrgico;
paciente *m* (enfermo *m*) de cirugía
i malato *m* chirurgico;
malato *m* di chirurgia
n chirurgische patiënt;
operatiepatiënt
d chirurgischer Patient *m* (Kranker *m*)

2196 SURGICAL PERSONNEL;
SURGICAL STAFF
f personnel *m* chirurgical
e personal *m* quirúrgico
i personale *m* chirurgico
n chirurgisch personeel *n*
d chirurgisches Personal *n*

2197 SURGICAL SPECIALITY
f spécialité *f* chirurgicale
e especialidad *f* quirúrgica
i specialità *f* chirurgica
n chirurgisch specialisme *n*
d chirurgische Spezialität *f*

2198 SURGICAL STAFF
see: SURGICAL PERSONNEL

2199 SURGICAL SUITE
see: OPERATING BLOCK

2200 SURGICAL UNIT
see: SURGERY UNIT

2201 SYNDROME
see: CLINICAL PICTURE

T

2202 TEACHING HOSPITAL
see: ACADEMIC HOSPITAL

2203 TEACHING NURSE
f infirmière *f* enseignante
e enfermera *f* docente
i infermiera *f* istruttrice
n docent-verpleegkundige; verpleegkundig docent
d Unterrichtsschwester *f*; Lehrschwester *f*; Schulschwester *f*

2204 TEAM CARE NURSE; TEAM NURSE
f infirmière *f* de groupe
e enfermera *f* de equipo
i infermiera *f* di gruppo
n teamverpleegster; teamverpleegkundige; teamverplegende
d Gruppenschwester *f*

2205 TEAM NURSE
see: TEAM CARE NURSE

2206 TEAM NURSING
see: GROUP NURSING

2207 TEAM NURSING CARE
see: GROUP NURSING

2208 TEMPERATURE CHART
f feuille *f* de température
e hoja *f* de temperatura
i cartellino *m* della temperatura
n temperatuurstaat; temperatuurlijst
d Fieberblatt *n*

2209 TERMINAL CARE
f soins *mpl* aux malades (patients) mourants
e cuidado *m* de los pacientes (enfermos) moribundos
i cure *fpl* ai malati moribondi
n terminale zorg
d Pflege *f* sterbender Patienten (Kranker)

2210 TERMINAL CARE DEPARTMENT; TERMINAL DEPARTMENT
f service *m* (département *m*) pour malades (patients) mourants
e servicio *m* (departamento *m*) para pacientes (enfermos) moribundos
i servizio *m* per malati moribondi
n afdeling voor terminale patiënten
d Abteilung *f* für sterbende Patienten (Kranke)

2211 TERMINAL CARE PATIENT
see: DYING PATIENT

2212 TERMINAL CARE UNIT; TERMINAL UNIT
f unité *f* pour malades (patients) mourants
e unidad *f* para pacientes (enfermos) moribundos
i unità *f* per malati moribondi
n eenheid voor terminale patiënten
d Station *f* für sterbende Patienten (Kranke)

2213 TERMINAL DEPARTMENT
see: TERMINAL CARE DEPARTMENT

2214 TERMINAL PATIENT
see: DYING PATIENT

2215 TERMINAL UNIT
see: TERMINAL CARE UNIT

2216 THALASSOTHERAPY
see: MARINE THERAPY

2217 THEATRE CLOTHING
see: OPERATING ROOM CLOTHING

2218 THEATRE LINEN
see: OPERATING ROOM LINEN

2219 THEATRE NURSE
see: OPERATING ROOM NURSE

2220 THEATRE NURSING
see: OPERATING ROOM NURSING

2221 THEATRE SISTER
see: OPERATING ROOM SISTER

2222 THEATRE STERILE STORE
f dépôt *m* de matériel d'opération stérile
e almacén *m* de material de operación estéril
i deposito *m* del materiale sterilizzato operatorio
n berging voor steriel operatiemateriaal
d Lager *n* für steriles Operationsmaterial

2223 THERAPEUTIC COMMUNITY
f communauté *f* thérapeutique; collectivité *f* thérapeutique
e comunidad *f* terapéutica
i comunità *f* terapeutica; collettività *f* terapeutica
n therapeutische gemeenschap; therapeutisch milieu *n*
d therapeutische Gemeinschaft *f*

2224 THERAPEUTIC RADIOLOGY
f radiologie *f* thérapeutique
e radiología *f* terapéutica
i radiologia *f* terapeutica
n therapeutische radiologie
d therapeutische Radiologie *f*

2225 THERAPEUTICS; THERAPY
f thérapeutique *f*; thérapie *f*
e terapéutica *f*; terapia *f*
i terapeutica *f*; terapia *f*
n therapie
d Therapie *f*

2226 THERAPEUTICS DEPARTMENT; THERAPY DEPARTMENT
f service *m* (département *m*) de thérapeutique; service *m* (département *m*) de thérapie

e servicio *m* (departamento *m*) de terapéutica;
servicio *m* (departamento *m*) de terapia
i servizio *m* di terapeutica;
servizio *m* di terapia
n therapie-afdeling
d Therapieabteilung *f*

2227 THERAPEUTIST;
THERAPIST
f thérapeute *m*
e terapeuta *m*
i terapeuta *m*;
terapista *m*
n therapeut
d Therapeut *m*;
Heilkundiger *m*

2228 THERAPIST
see: THERAPEUTIST

2229 THERAPY
see: THERAPEUTICS

2230 THERAPY DEPARTMENT
see: THERAPEUTICS DEPARTMENT

2231 THORACIC SURGEON
f chirurgien *m* thoracique
e cirujano *m* torácico
i chirurgo *m* toracico
n thoraxchirurg
d Thoraxchirurg *m*

2232 THORACIC SURGERY
f chirurgie *f* thoracique
e cirugía *f* torácica
i chirurgia *f* toracica
n thoraxchirurgie
d Thoraxchirurgie *f*

2233 THORACIC SURGERY DEPARTMENT
f service *m* (département *m*) de chirurgie thoracique
e servicio *m* (departamento *m*) de cirugía torácica
i divisione *f* di chirurgia toracica
n afdeling voor thoraxchirurgie
d Abteilung *f* für Thoraxchirurgie

2234 THORACIC SURGERY UNIT
f unité *f* de chirurgie thoracique
e unidad *f* de cirugía torácica
i unità *f* di chirurgia toracica
n eenheid voor thoraxchirurgie
d Station *f* für Thoraxchirurgie

2235 TISSUE BANK
f banque *f* des tissus
e banco *m* de tejidos
i banca *f* dei tessuti
n weefselbank
d Gewebebank *f*

2236 TONSILLECTOMY ROOM
f salle *f* d'amygdalectomie
e sala *f* de tonsilectomía
i sala *f* di tonsillectomia
n sluderkamer
d Raum *m* für Amygdalektomie

2237 TOXICOLOGIST
f toxicologue *m*
e toxicólogo *m*
i tossicologo *m*
n toxicoloog
d Toxikologe *m*

2238 TOXICOLOGY
f toxicologie *f*
e toxicología *f*
i tossicologia *f*
n toxicologie
d Toxikologie *f*

2239 TRAFFIC ACCIDENT SERVICE
f service *m* de secours aux victimes de la circulation
e servicio *m* de accidentes de circulación;
servicio *m* de atropellos
i servizio *m* di pronto soccorso alle vittime degli incidenti stradali
n verkeersongevallendienst
d Verkehrsunfalldienst *m*

2240 TRAFFIC MEDICINE
f médecine *f* de la circulation
e medicina *f* de circulación;
medicina *f* de tráfico
i medicina *f* del traffico
n verkeersgeneeskunde
d Verkehrsmedizin *f*

2241 TRAINING SCHOOL FOR MIDWIVES
f école *f* pour accoucheuses
e escuela *f* para parteras
i scuola *f* di levatrice
n school voor vroedvrouwen
d Hebammenschule *f*

2242 TRAINING SCHOOL FOR NURSES
see: NURSES' SCHOOL

2243 TRANSPLANTATION
f transplantation *f*;
greffe *f*
e trasplante *m*
i trapianto *m*
n transplantatie
d Transplantation *f*;
Überpflanzung *f*

2244 TRANSPLANTATION SURGERY
f chirurgie *f* de transplantation
e cirugía *f* de trasplante
i chirurgia *f* dei trapianti
n transplantatiechirurgie
d Transplantationschirurgie *f*

2245 TRANSPLANTATION SURGERY DEPARTMENT
f service *m* (département *m*) de chirurgie de transplantation
e servicio *m* (departamento *m*) de cirugía de trasplante
i servizio *m* di chirurgia dei trapianti
n afdeling voor transplantatiechirurgie
d Abteilung *f* für Transplantationschirurgie

2246 TRANSPLANTATION SURGERY HOSPITAL
f hôpital *m* de chirurgie de transplantation
e hospital *m* de cirugía de trasplante
i ospedale *m* di chirurgia dei trapianti
n ziekenhuis *n* voor transplantatiechirurgie
d Krankenhaus *n* für Transplantationschirurgie

2247 TRANSPLANTATION SURGERY UNIT
f unité *f* de chirurgie de transplantation

e unidad *f* de cirugía de trasplante
i unità *f* di chirurgia dei trapianti
n eenheid voor transplantatiechirurgie
d Station *f* für Transplantationschirurgie

2248 TRANSPLANT BANK
f banque *f* d'organes
e banco *m* de órganos
i banca *f* d'organi
n orgaanbank
d Transplantationsbank *f*

2249 TRAUMA CENTRE (CENTER)
f centre *m* traumatologique;
centre *m* de traumatologie
e centro *m* traumatológico;
centro *m* de traumatología
i centro *m* traumatologico;
centro *m* di traumatologia
n traumatologisch centrum *n*
d traumatologisches Zentrum *n*

2250 TRAUMATOLOGY
f traumatologie *f*
e traumatología *f*
i traumatologia *f*
n traumatologie
d Traumatologie *f*

2251 TREATMENT
f traitement *m*
e tratamiento *m*
i trattamento *m*
n behandeling
d Behandlung *f*

2252 TREATMENT BLOCK
see: MEDICAL BLOCK

2253 TREATMENT CHART
f feuille *f* d'observation
e hoja *f* de observación
i foglio *m* d'osservazione
n behandelingskaart
d Beobachtungsbogen *m*

2254 TREATMENT COSTS
f coûts *mpl* de traitement
e gastos *mpl* de tratamiento
i costi *mpl* del trattamento;
spese *fpl* per il trattamento
n behandelingskosten
d Behandlungskosten *pl*

2255 TREATMENT DEPARTMENT
f service *m* (département *m*) de traitement
e servicio *m* (departamento *m*) de tratamiento
i servizio *m* di trattamento
n nevenafdeling;
behandelafdeling
d Behandlungsabteilung *f*

2256 TREATMENT DURATION
f durée *f* de traitement
e duración *f* del tratamiento
i durata *f* del trattamento
n behandelingsduur
d Behandlungsdauer *f*

2257 TREATMENT POOL
see: EXERCISE POOL

2258 TREATMENT ROOM
f salle *f* de traitement
e sala *f* de tratamiento
i sala *f* di trattamento
n behandelruimte;
behandelkamer
d Behandlungsraum *m*;
Behandlungszimmer *n*

2259 TROPICAL DISEASE
f maladie *f* tropicale
e enfermedad *f* tropical
i malattia *f* tropicale
n tropische ziekte
d Tropenkrankheit *f*

2260 TROPICAL DISEASES HOSPITAL
f hôpital *m* pour maladies tropicales
e hospital *m* para enfermedades tropicales
i ospedale *m* per malattie tropicali
n ziekenhuis *n* voor tropische ziekten
d Krankenhaus *n* für Tropenkrankheiten

2261 TROPICAL MEDICINE
f médecine *f* tropicale
e medicina *f* tropical
i medicina *f* tropicale
n tropische geneeskunde
d Tropenmedizin *f*

2262 TUBERCULOSIS CARE
f soins *mpl* aux tuberculeux
e cuidado *m* de los tuberculosos
i cure *fpl* ai tubercolotici
n zorg voor tuberculosepatiënten
d Betreuung *f* von Tuberkulosepatienten

2263 TUBERCULOSIS CENTRE (CENTER)
f centre *m* antituberculeux;
centre *m* pour tuberculeux
e centro *m* antituberculoso;
preventorio *m* antituberculoso
i centro *m* antitubercolare;
centro *m* per tubercolotici
n consultatiebureau *n* voor tuberculosebestrijding
d Tuberkulosezentrum *n*

2264 TUBERCULOSIS CONTROL
f lutte *f* antituberculeuse;
lutte *f* contre la tuberculose
e lucha *f* antituberculosa
i lotta *f* antitubercolare;
lotta *f* contro la tubercolosi
n tuberculosebestrijding
d Tuberkulosebekämpfung *f*

2265 TUBERCULOSIS HOSPITAL
f hôpital *m* antituberculeux;
hôpital *m* pour tuberculeux;

établissement *m* antituberculeux;
établissement *m* pour tuberculeux
e hospital *m* antituberculoso;
hospital *m* para tuberculosis
i ospedale *m* antitubercolare;
ospedale *m* per tubercolotici
n ziekenhuis *n* voor tuberculosepatiënten
d Tuberkulosekrankenhaus *n*

2266 TUBERCULOSIS LABORATORY
f laboratoire *m* de tuberculose
e laboratorio *m* de tuberculosis
i laboratorio *m* di tubercolosi
n tuberculoselaboratorium *n*
d Tuberkuloselaboratorium *n*

2267 TUBERCULOSIS NURSING
f soins *mpl* infirmiers aux tuberculeux
e enfermería *f* de los tuberculosos
i cure *fpl* infermieristiche ai tubercolotici
n verpleging van tuberculosepatiënten
d Pflege *f* von Tuberkulosepatienten

2268 TUBERCULOSIS SANATORIUM
f sanatorium *m* antituberculeux;
sanatorium *m* pour tuberculeux
e sanatorio *m* antituberculoso;
sanatorio *m* para tuberculosis
i sanatorio *m* antitubercolare;
sanatorio *m* per tubercolotici
n sanatorium *n* voor tuberculosepatiënten
d Tuberkulosesanatorium *n*;
Tuberkuloseheilstätte *f*

2269 TUBERCULOSIS SERVICES
f services *mpl* de lutte antituberculeuse
e servicios *mpl* antituberculosos
i servizi *mpl* di lotta contro la tubercolosi
n tuberculosediensten
d Tuberkulosedienste *mpl*

2270 TURNOVER INTERVAL
f intervalle *m* de rotation
e intervalo *m* de ingresos;
intermitencia *f* de ingresos
i intervallo *m* di rotazione
n doorstromingsinterval *n*
d Durchgangsintervall *n*

2271 TURNOVER PER BED
f rotation *f* par lit
e ingresos *mpl* por cama
i rotazione *f* per letto
n doorstroming per bed
d Durchgang *m* pro Bett

2272 TYPE OF ACCOMODATION
f classe *f* d'hospitalisation
e clase *f* de hospitalización
i classe *f* d'ospedalizzazione
n verpleegklasse
d Pflegeklasse *f*

2273 TYPE OF NURSING CARE
f régime *m* de soins infirmiers
e régimen *m* de enfermería
i regime *m* di cure infermieristiche
n verpleegwijze
d Pflegeform *f*;
Pflegeart *f*

U

2274 ULTRASONIC APPARATUS
f appareils *mpl* par ultrasons
e aparatos *mpl* ultrasonoros
i apparecchi *mpl* ad ultrasuoni
n ultrasonische apparatuur
d Ultraschallgeräte *npl*

2275 ULTRASONIC THERAPY
f thérapie *f* par ultrasons
e terapia *f* ultrasonora
i terapia *f* ad ultrasuoni
n ultrasonische therapie
d Ultraschalltherapie *f*

2276 UNIT BATH
f bain *m* d'unité
e baño *m* de unidad
i bagno *m* d'unità
n afdelingsbad *n*
d Stationsbad *n*

2277 UNIVERSITY CLINIC
f clinique *f* universitaire
e clínica *f* universitaria
i clinica *f* universitaria
n universiteitskliniek
d Universitätsklinik *f*;
Universitätsklinikum *n*

2278 UNIVERSITY HEALTH CARE SERVICES;
UNIVERSITY HEALTH SERVICES
f services *mpl* sanitaires universitaires
e servicios *mpl* sanitarios universitarios
i servizi *mpl* sanitari universitari
n universitaire gezondheidsdiensten
d Universitätsgesundheitsfürsorgedienste *mpl*

2279 UNIVERSITY HEALTH SERVICES
see: UNIVERSITY HEALTH CARE SERVICES

2280 UNIVERSITY HOSPITAL
see: ACADEMIC HOSPITAL

2281 UNIVERSITY MENTAL HEALTH CLINIC;
UNIVERSITY PSYCHIATRIC CLINIC
f clinique *f* de santé mentale universitaire;
clinique *f* psychiatrique universitaire
e clínica *f* de salud mental universitaria;
clínica *f* psiquiátrica universitaria
i clinica *f* psichiatrica universitaria
n universitaire psychiatrische kliniek
d Universitätsklinik *f* für Psychiatrie

2282 UNIVERSITY PSYCHIATRIC CLINIC
see: UNIVERSITY MENTAL HEALTH CLINIC

2283 URBAN HEALTH CARE FACILITIES;
URBAN HEALTH CARE SERVICES;
URBAN HEALTH FACILITIES;
URBAN HEALTH SERVICES
f services *mpl* sanitaires urbains
e servicios *mpl* sanitarios urbanos
i servizi *mpl* sanitari urbani
n stedelijke gezondheidsdiensten
d städtische Gesundheitsdienste *mpl*

2284 URBAN HEALTH CARE SERVICES
see: URBAN HEALTH CARE FACILITIES

2285 URBAN HEALTH FACILITIES
see: URBAN HEALTH CARE FACILITIES

2286 URBAN HEALTH SERVICES
see: URBAN HEALTH CARE FACILITIES

2287 URBAN HOSPITAL
see: CITY HOSPITAL

2288 URINAL
f urinal *m*
e orinal *m*
i orinale *m*
n urinaal *n*
d Urinal *n*

2289 URINE ANALYSIS
f analyse *f* d'urine
e análisis *m* y *f* de orina;
uroscopia *f*
i analisi *f* dell'orina
n urine-onderzoek *n*
d Urinanalyse *f*

2290 UROLOGICAL CLINIC;
UROLOGY CLINIC
f clinique *f* urologique;
clinique *f* d'urologie
e clínica *f* urológica;
clínica *f* de urología
i clinica *f* urologica;
clinica *f* d'urologia
n urologische kliniek
d urologische Klinik *f*

2291 UROLOGICAL DEPARTMENT;
UROLOGY DEPARTMENT
f service *m* (département *m*) urologique;
service *m* (département *m*) d'urologie
e servicio *m* (departamento *m*) urológico;
servicio *m* (departamento *m*) de urología
i divisione *f* urologica;
divisione *f* d'urologia
n urologische afdeling
d urologische Abteilung *f*

2292 UROLOGICAL HOSPITAL;
UROLOGY HOSPITAL
f hôpital *m* urologique;
hôpital *m* d'urologie
e hospital *m* urológico;
hospital *m* de urología
i ospedale *m* urologico;
ospedale *m* d'urologia

n urologisch ziekenhuis *n*
d urologisches Krankenhaus *n*

2293 UROLOGICAL UNIT;
UROLOGY UNIT
f unité *f* urologique;
unité *f* d'urologie
e unidad *f* urológica;
unidad *f* de urología
i unità *f* urologica;
unità *f* d'urologia
n urologische eenheid
d urologische Station *f*

2294 UROLOGIST
f urologue *m*
e urólogo *m*
i urologo *m*
n uroloog
d Urologe *m*

2295 UROLOGY
f urologie *f*
e urología *f*
i urologia *f*
n urologie
d Urologie *f*

2296 UROLOGY CLINIC
see: UROLOGICAL CLINIC

2297 UROLOGY DEPARTMENT
see: UROLOGICAL DEPARTMENT

2298 UROLOGY HOSPITAL
see: UROLOGICAL HOSPITAL

2299 UROLOGY UNIT
see: UROLOGICAL UNIT

V

2300 VACCINATION
f vaccination *f*
e vacunación *f*
i vaccinazione *f*
n vaccinatie
d Impfung *f*;
Schutzimpfung *f*

2301 VACCINATION CERTIFICATE;
VACCINATION PAPER
f certificat *m* de vaccination
e certificado *m* de vacunación
i certificato *m* di vaccinazione
n vaccinatiebewijs *n*
d Impfschein *m*

2302 VACCINATION PAPER
see: VACCINATION CERTIFICATE

2303 VACCINATOR
f vaccinateur *m*
e vacunador *m*
i vaccinatore *m*
n vaccinator
d Impfer *m*

2304 VENERAL DISEASE
f maladie *f* vénérienne
e venéreo *m*
i malattia *f* venerea
n geslachtsziekte
d Geschlechtskrankheit *f*

2305 VENERAL DISEASES CLINIC
f clinique *f* de maladies vénériennes
e clínica *f* de venéreos
i clinica *f* dermosifilopatica;
clinica *f* di dermosifilopatia
n kliniek voor geslachtsziekten
d Klinik *f* für Geschlechtskrankheiten

2306 VENERAL DISEASES DEPARTMENT
f service *m* (département *m*) de maladies vénériennes
e servicio *m* (departamento *m*) de venéreos
i divisione *f* dermosifilopatica;
divisione *f* di dermosifilopatia
n afdeling voor geslachtsziekten
d Abteilung *f* für Geschlechtskrankheiten

2307 VENERAL DISEASES HOSPITAL
f hôpital *m* de maladies vénériennes
e hospital *m* de venéreos
i ospedale *m* dermosifilopatico;
ospedale *m* di dermosifilopatia
n ziekenhuis *n* voor geslachtsziekten
d Krankenhaus *n* für Geschlechtskrankheiten

2308 VENERAL DISEASES UNIT
f unité *f* de maladies vénériennes
e unidad *f* de venéreos
i unità *f* dermosifilopatica;
unità *f* di dermosifilopatia
n eenheid voor geslachtsziekten
d Station *f* für Geschlechtskrankheiten

2309 VERMIN CONTROL
see: INSECT CONTROL

2310 VIROLOGY LABORATORY
f laboratoire *m* virologique;
laboratoire *m* de virologie
e laboratorio *m* virológico;
laboratorio *m* de virología
i laboratorio *m* virologico;
laboratorio *m* di virologia
n virologisch laboratorium *n*
d virologisches Laboratorium *n*

2311 VISITING HOURS;
VISITING TIME
f heures *fpl* de visite;
horaire *m* de visite
e horas *fpl* de visita
i orario *m* di visita
n bezoekuren;
bezoektijd
d Besuchszeit *f*

2312 VISITING NURSE
see: DISTRICT NURSE

2313 VISITING TIME
see: VISITING HOURS

2314 VISITORS' WAITING ROOM
f salle *f* d'attente des visiteurs
e sala *f* de espera para visitantes
i sala *f* d'attesa dei visitatori
n wachtkamer voor bezoekers
d Warteraum *m* für Besucher;
Wartezimmer *n* für Besucher

2315 VISIT PAID TO A PATIENT
f visite *f* rendue à un malade
e visita *f* de enfermo
i visita *f* resa ad un malato
n ziekenbezoek *n*
d Krankenbesuch *m*

2316 VOCATIONAL REHABILITATION
see: PROFESSIONAL REHABILITATION

2317 VOLUNTARY ADMISSION
f admission *f* libre
e admisión *f* voluntaria
i ricovero *m* volontario
n vrijwillige opname
d freiwillige Aufnahme *f*

2318 VOLUNTARY HEALTH CARE INSURANCE;
VOLUNTARY HEALTH INSURANCE
f assurance-maladie *f* volontaire

e seguro *m* de salud voluntario;
seguro *m* de enfermedad voluntario
i assicurazione *f* malattia volontaria;
assicurazione *f* contro le malattie volontaria
n vrijwillige ziekte(kosten)verzekering
d freiwillige Krankenversicherung *f*

2319 VOLUNTARY HEALTH INSURANCE
see: VOLUNTARY HEALTH CARE INSURANCE

2320 VOLUNTARY INSURED PERSON
f assuré *m* volontaire
e asegurado *m* voluntario
i assicurato *m* volontario
n vrijwillig verzekerde
d freiwillig Versicherter *m*

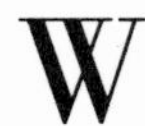

2321 WAITING ROOM
f salle *f* d'attente
e sala *f* de espera
i sala *f* d'attesa
n wachtkamer
d Warteraum *m*; Wartezimmer *m*

2322 WAITING TIME
f temps *m* d'attente
e tiempo *m* de espera
i tempo *m* di attesa
n wachttijd
d Wartezeit *f*

2323 WARD CHIEF NURSE; WARD HEAD NURSE; WARD SISTER
f infirmière -chef *f* de salle
e enfermera *f* jefe de sala; jefe *f* de sala
i infermiera-capo *f* sala; capo-sala *f*
n zaalhoofd *n*
d Saaloberschwester *f*

2324 WARD HEAD NURSE
see: WARD CHIEF NURSE

2325 WARD KITCHEN
see: FLOORKITCHEN

2326 WARD NURSING; WARD NURSING CARE
f soins *mpl* infirmiers en salle
e enfermería *f* en sala
i cure *fpl* infermieristiche in sala
n zaalverpleging
d Saalpflege *f*

2327 WARD NURSING CARE
see: WARD NURSING

2328 WARD ROOM
see: PATIENT ROOM

2329 WARD SISTER
see: WARD CHIEF NURSE

2330 WATER BED
f lit *m* d'eau
e cama *f* de agua
i letto *m* d'acqua
n waterbed *n*
d Wasserbett *n*

2331 WAX BATH
f bain *m* de paraffine
e baño *m* de parafina
i bagno *m* di paraffina
n paraffinebad *n*
d Paraffinbad *n*

2332 WEEKEND CENTRE (CENTER)
f centre *m* de fin de semaine
e centro *m* de fin de semana
i centro *m* di fine settimana
n weekeinde-centrum *n*
d Wochenendezentrum *n*

2333 WEEKEND HOSPITAL
f hôpital *m* de fin de semaine
e hospital *m* de fin de semana
i ospedale *m* di fine settimana
n weekeinde-ziekenhuis *n*
d Wochenendekrankenhaus *n*

2334 WEEKEND PSYCHIATRIC CARE
f soins *mpl* psychiatriques de fin de semaine
e cuidado *m* psiquiátrico de fin de semana
i cure *fpl* psichiatriche di fine settimana
n psychiatrische zorg in het weekeinde
d psychiatrische Fürsorge *f* im Wochenende

2335 WHIRLPOOL BATH
f douches *fpl* sous-marines
e baño *m* con torbellino de agua
i doccie *fpl* sottomarine
n whirlpoolbad *n*
d Bad *n* mit Wasserwirblung

2336 WHO
see: WORLD HEALTH ORGANIZATION

2337 WOMEN'S CLINIC
see: GYNECOLOGICAL CLINIC

2338 WOMEN'S DEPARTMENT
see: GYNECOLOGICAL DEPARTMENT

2339 WOMEN'S HOSPITAL
see: GYNECOLOGICAL DEPARTMENT

2340 WOMEN'S UNIT
see: GYNECOLOGICAL UNIT

2341 WORK DISABLEMENT
f incapacité *f* de travail
e ineptitud *f* para el trabajo; incapacidad *f* para el trabajo
i inabilità *f* al lavoro
n arbeidsongeschiktheid
d Arbeitsunfähigkeit *f*

2342 WORK THERAP(EUT)IST
see: ERGOTHERAPEUTIST

2343 WORK THERAPY
see: ERGOTHERAPY

2344 WORK THERAPY DEPARTMENT
see: ERGOTHERAPY DEPARTMENT

2345 WORLD HEALTH
f santé *f* mondiale

e salud *f* mundial
i sanità *f* mondiale
n wereldgezondheid
d Weltgesundheit *f*

2346 WORLD HEALTH ORGANIZATION;
WHO
f Organisation *f* Mondiale de la Santé;
OMS *f*
e Organización *f* Mundial de la Salud;
OMS *f*
i Organizzazione *f* Mondiale della Sanità;
OMS *f*
n Wereldgezondheidsorganisatie;
WGO
d Weltgesundheitsorganisation *f*;
WGO *f*

X

2347 X-RAY APPARATUS
see: RADIOLOGICAL APPARATUS

2348 X-RAY DEPARTMENT
see: RADIOLOGICAL DEPARTMENT

2349 X-RAY EXAMINATION
see: RADIOGRAPHY

2350 X-RAY FILM
f film *m* radiologique;
film *m* radiographique
e película *f* radiológica;
película *f* de rayos x
i film *m* radiologico;
lastra *f* radiologica
n röntgenfilm
d Röntgenfilm *m*

2351 X-RAY FILM ARCHIVES;
X-RAY FILM STORE
f dépôt *m* pour films radiologiques
e archivo *m* de películas radiológicas
i deposito *m* dei films radiologici;
archivio *m* radiografico
n röntgenarchief *n*;
berging voor röntgenfilms
d Röntgenarchiv *n*;
Lager *n* für Röntgenfilme

2352 X-RAY FILM STORE
see: X-RAY FILM ARCHIVES

2353 X-RAY PERSONNEL
see: RADIOLOGICAL PERSONNEL

2354 X-RAY PICTURE
see: RADIOGRAPH

2355 X-RAY PROTECTION
f protection *f* contre les rayons x
e protección *f* contra los rayos x
i protezione *f* contro i raggi x
n bescherming tegen röntgenstralen
d Röntgenstrahlenschutz *m*

2356 X-RAY ROOM
see: RADIOLOGICAL ROOM

2357 X-RAY STAFF
see: RADIOLOGICAL PERSONNEL

2358 X-RAY TECHNOLOGY
see: RADIOLOGICAL TECHNOLOGY

2359 X-RAY THERAP(EUT)IST
see: RADIOTHERAPEUTIST

2360 X-RAY THERAPY
see: RADIOTHERAPY

2361 X-RAY UNIT
see: RADIOLOGICAL UNIT

2362 X-RAY VIEWING ROOM
f salle *f* d'examen des clichés
e sala *f* para lectura de radiografías
i sala *f* d'esame delle lastre
n fotobekijkkamer
d Schauraum *m* für Röntgenaufnahmen

Y

2363 YOUTH HEALTH CARE
f soins *mpl* sanitaires de la jeunesse
e cuidado *m* sanitario de la juventud
i assistenza *f* sanitaria della gioventù
n jeugdgezondheidszorg
d Jugendgesundheitsfürsorge *f*

FRANÇAIS

ESPAÑOL

ITALIANO

NEDERLANDS

DEUTSCH